The Vaping Controversy

**Recent Titles in
21st-Century Turning Points**

The Vaping Controversy

Laurie Collier Hillstrom

21st-Century Turning Points

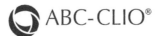

An Imprint of ABC-CLIO, LLC

Santa Barbara, California • Denver, Colorado

Library of Congress Cataloging in Publication Control Number: 2019019269

ISBN: 978-1-4408-7110-8 (print)
    978-1-4408-7111-5 (ebook)

23 22 21 20 19   1 2 3 4 5

This book is also available as an eBook.

ABC-CLIO
An Imprint of ABC-CLIO, LLC

ABC-CLIO, LLC
147 Castilian Drive
Santa Barbara, California 93117
www.abc-clio.com

This book is printed on acid-free paper ∞

Manufactured in the United States of America

Contents

Series Foreword

21st-Century Turning Points is a general reference series that has been crafted for use by high school and undergraduate students as well as members of the general public. The purpose of the series is to give readers a clear, authoritative, and unbiased understanding of major fast-breaking events, movements, people, and issues that are transforming American life, culture, and politics in this turbulent new century. Each volume constitutes a one-stop resource for learning about a single issue or event currently dominating America's news headlines and political discussions—issues or events that, in many cases, are also driving national debate about our country's leaders, institutions, values, and priorities.

Each volume in the *21st-Century Turning Points* series begins with an **Overview** of the event or issue that is the subject of the book. It then provides a suite of informative chronologically arranged narrative entries on specific **Landmarks** in the evolution of the event or issue in question. This section provides both vital historical context and insights into present-day news events to give readers a full and clear understanding of how current issues and controversies evolved.

The next section of the book is devoted to examining the **Impacts** of the event or issue in question on various aspects of American life, including political, economic, cultural, and interpersonal implications. It is followed by a chapter of biographical **Profiles** that summarize the life experiences and personal beliefs of prominent individuals associated with the event or issue in question.

Finally, each book concludes with a topically-organized **Further Resources** list of important and informative resources—from influential books to fascinating websites—to which readers can turn for additional information, and a carefully compiled subject **Index**.

These complementary elements, found in every book in the series, work together to create an evenhanded, authoritative, and user-friendly tool for gaining a deeper and more accurate understanding of the fast-changing nation in which we live—and the issues and moments that define us as we move deeper into the twenty-first century.

CHAPTER ONE

Overview of the Vaping Controversy

Electronic cigarettes—also known as e-cigarettes, e-cigs, vapes, vape pens, mods, and electronic nicotine delivery systems (ENDS)—first appeared in the United States around 2007. A decade later, more than 10 million American adults—plus 3.6 million young people under age 18—had taken up vaping. The rapid adoption of this new, relatively untested technology, and especially its exploding popularity among teenagers, raised concerns about the potential impact of vaping on public health.

E-cigarettes work by using a battery-powered heating coil or atomizer to heat a liquid solution—known as e-liquid, e-juice, or vape juice—and turn it into an inhalable vapor. Depending on the type of e-cigarette, e-liquids come in disposable cartridges or pods, as well as refillable tanks. Most e-liquids contain nicotine—a chemical stimulant derived from the tobacco plant—along with water, flavoring, and common food additives such as propylene glycol and vegetable glycerin. Inhaling vapor from an e-cigarette, known as vaping, delivers nicotine through the lungs and bloodstream to the brain, giving users a similar sensation to smoking a cigarette.

Proponents of vaping claim that e-cigarettes offer a safer means of nicotine delivery than traditional cigarettes. They argue that the health risks of cigarette smoking come from burning tobacco, which releases toxic chemicals into smokers' lungs and the surrounding air. E-cigarettes, in contrast, do not involve combustion and do not produce smoke. Instead, they produce an aerosol vapor that is similar to the theatrical fog used in the entertainment industry. Many vaping enthusiasts are former cigarette smokers who succeeded in quitting, often after numerous previous attempts, by switching to e-cigarettes. Some offer glowing testimonials about the health improvements they experience by vaping instead of smoking.

Pro-vaping advocates characterize concerns about the safety of e-cigarettes as unwarranted and overblown, especially considering that the alternative for many adult vapers is smoking cigarettes, which causes the premature death of half a million Americans every year. They portray e-cigarettes as valuable tools for tobacco harm reduction and smoking cessation, and they strenuously resist efforts to regulate e-cigarettes and restrict vaping rights. David Sweanor, a professor of health policy at the University of Ottawa, described the lifesaving potential of e-cigarettes as "something that would rival the eradication of smallpox" (Gross 2017).

On the other side of the vaping debate are public health officials and tobacco-control advocates, some of whom spent decades fighting to reduce the prevalence of cigarette smoking and smoking-related diseases in the United States. Antismoking campaigns contributed to a steady decline in adult cigarette smoking rates to an all-time low of 14 percent in 2017 (CDC 2018). Around the same time, though, the popularity of e-cigarettes exploded, and vaping rates exceeded 20 percent among high-school students in 2018 (Cullen et al. 2018). Critics claim that e-cigarette manufacturers intentionally target young people with sweet, fruity flavors and colorful social media campaigns that promote vaping as exciting, glamorous, edgy, and cool.

Although public health researchers generally consider e-cigarettes less harmful than combustible cigarettes, they stress that the long-term health risks of vaping remain unknown. "Some people say these risks are very, very low, but our question is 'how low?'" said Armando Peruga, a tobacco-control expert with the World Health Organization (WHO). "If smoking a cigarette is like jumping from the 100th floor, using an e-cigarette is certainly like jumping from a lower floor, but which floor? We don't know" (Fleck 2014). Some studies have found toxic chemicals in e-cigarette vapor or in the urine of vapers. Other studies cast doubt on claims that e-cigarettes help people quit smoking. Instead, research suggests that many vapers continue using traditional, "combustible" cigarettes, despite indications that such "dual use" may be more dangerous than either smoking or vaping alone.

The main concern expressed by public health officials and antismoking organizations centers on youth vaping. They assert that e-cigarette use is exposing a new generation of Americans to nicotine, putting them at risk for lifelong physical dependency or addiction. Nicotine poses particular hazards for young people because it permanently affects the reward circuits in developing brains, increasing the likelihood that young vapers will smoke cigarettes or seek stimulation from other drugs, such as marijuana, cocaine, and methamphetamine. Critics note that one tiny pod of e-liquid for the popular Juul brand e-cigarette contains as much nicotine as a pack of cigarettes, yet the majority of underage users do not realize that vaping products contain nicotine at all. "If you were to design your ideal nicotine-delivery device to addict large numbers of United States kids, you'd invent Juul," said pediatric tobacco expert Jonathan Winickoff (Tolentino 2018). Many teenagers perceive vaping as harmless fun, which leads to e-cigarette use among kids who never would have considered smoking cigarettes. Across the country, teachers and administrators report students hiding e-cigarettes in their pockets, purses, or backpacks and vaping in school bathrooms, hallways, classrooms, parking lots, and buses.

Alarmed by the rapid increase in e-cigarette use among teenagers, tobacco-control activists demanded that the U.S. Food and Drug Administration (FDA) subject vaping products to the same regulations as combustible cigarettes. In 2018, then-FDA Commissioner Scott Gottlieb threatened to remove popular vaping products from the market if e-cigarette manufacturers failed to cooperate with the FDA to combat what he described as an "epidemic" of youth vaping. Pro-vaping advocates fought against the proposed regulations, arguing that restricting the availability of e-cigarettes and flavored e-liquids would harm public health by pushing adults back to traditional cigarettes. The national debate grew even more polarized as large tobacco companies increased their involvement in the vaping industry.

The Tobacco Industry and Tobacco Control Efforts

Tobacco is a plant in the nightshade family, along with bell peppers, tomatoes, and eggplant. Tobacco grows naturally in North America, and Native Americans used it for medicinal and religious purposes for thousands of years. European settlers established the first companies dedicated to cultivating, drying, and trading tobacco in the late 1700s. Cigarettes and cigars replaced chewing tobacco as the most popular tobacco products in the United States during the early twentieth century. Cigarette-smoking rates reached their highest point following World War II (1939–1945), driven by extensive advertising for such brands as Camel, Marlboro, Lucky Strike, and Pall Mall.

Public perceptions of cigarettes began to change in 1964, with the publication of the U.S Surgeon General's landmark report linking smoking to elevated risks of lung cancer, cardiovascular disease, and other health problems. Evidence also mounted about the addictive effects of nicotine, which cause physical cravings and withdrawal symptoms that make it extremely difficult for smokers to quit. As the American people learned about the harmful effects of smoking, antismoking groups pressured state and federal lawmakers to address the growing threat to public health. Over the next few years, Congress passed several laws aimed at discouraging cigarette smoking. The Federal Cigarette Labeling and Advertising Act of 1965 required tobacco companies to place a health warning label on cigarette packages, for instance, while the Public Health Cigarette Smoking Act of 1969 banned cigarette advertising from American radio and television broadcasts.

For many years, big tobacco companies such as Brown and Williamson, Philip Morris, and R. J. Reynolds used their vast financial resources and political influence to suppress information about smoking-related health risks, sow doubts about the link between tobacco use and disease, deny the addictive capacity of nicotine, and resist regulation of cigarette marketing and sales. It took concerted efforts by legislators, regulators, attorneys, activists, and whistleblowers to expose these deceptive practices and hold the tobacco industry accountable.

In the early 1990s, under the leadership of Commissioner David A. Kessler, the FDA uncovered evidence that tobacco manufacturers intentionally manipulated the levels of nicotine in cigarettes to increase their addictive potential and specifically targeted underage youth to create a new generation of smokers. In 1994, U.S. Representative Henry Waxman (D-CA) called the leaders of the seven largest tobacco companies to testify before Congress. When the executives swore under oath that nicotine was not addictive, the resulting public outrage led to new calls for federal regulation. The tobacco companies successfully claimed that cigarettes did not fall under the FDA's jurisdiction, however, because they were neither consumed as food nor administered as therapeutic drugs.

For decades, the cigarette makers avoided liability for selling a deadly product in countless lawsuits brought by individual smokers and their families. In 1994, though, a group of state attorneys general led by Mike Moore of Alabama employed a new legal strategy. They filed a class-action lawsuit accusing the tobacco companies of knowingly creating a public health crisis that forced the states to spend millions of extra dollars to treat smoking-related diseases through Medicaid and other health care programs. As the case proceeded, several whistleblowers came forward to

provide secret documents and inside information proving that the cigarette makers engaged in fraud and conspiracy to hide the dangers of their
product from the public. In 1998, the tobacco companies agreed to pay
the states $246 billion in compensation over 25 years as part of the largest
legal settlement in U.S. history. The agreement also required the cigarette
manufacturers to dissolve industry-funded groups that worked to conceal
the negative health effects of smoking, stop using marketing practices
designed to appeal to young people, and make 35 million pages of confidential corporate documents available to the public.

The 1990s and early 2000s also saw an increasing number of state and
local governments enact bans on smoking in public places. In 1992, the
U.S. Environmental Protection Agency (EPA) classified environmental
tobacco smoke as a human carcinogen, which launched a movement
aimed at protecting nonsmokers from the health risks of exposure to secondhand smoke. Early achievements included the creation of nonsmoking sections in restaurants and commercial airplanes. Antismoking
campaigns eventually resulted in the creation of smoke-free workplaces,
schools, and mass transit. By 2019, 28 states had enacted statewide bans
on smoking in all enclosed public places. Eleven states banned public
vaping as well (American Lung Association 2019).

In 2009, Congress finally granted the FDA authority to regulate the
content, manufacture, marketing, and sale of tobacco products by passing
the Family Smoking Prevention and Tobacco Control Act. The legislation
requires cigarette manufacturers to obtain FDA approval before introducing new tobacco products and to provide scientific evidence before making "modified risk" health claims. The Tobacco Control Act also increases
the size of warning labels, prohibits the use of cigarette flavorings other
than menthol, and includes several provisions aimed at reducing access to
tobacco products by underage youth.

Although lawsuits, regulations, and educational campaigns cut cigarette smoking rates in half since the release of the 1964 Surgeon General's
report, 42 million American adults and 3 million young people under 18
continued to smoke as of 2018, and smoking remained the leading cause
of preventable disease and death in the United States (U.S. Department of
Health and Human Services 2018). "Tobacco is, quite simply, in a league
of its own in terms of the sheer numbers and varieties of ways it kills and
maims people," said Thomas Frieden, former director of the U.S. Centers
for Disease Control and Prevention (Komaroff 2014). Although surveys
show that 70 percent of smokers want to quit—and more than 50 percent
attempt to do so each year—only 7 percent succeed, on average, due to
the addictive nature of nicotine (Truth Initiative 2018).

E-Cigarettes and Tobacco Harm Reduction

Electronic cigarettes originated as a form of tobacco harm reduction (THR). This public health strategy aims to lower the risks of nicotine use by encouraging smokers to switch from combustible cigarettes to less hazardous alternatives. The notion of improving smokers' lives motivated many of the people who contributed to the development of vaping technology. American inventor Herbert A. Gilbert, who received a U.S. patent on a device he called the "smokeless non-tobacco cigarette" in 1963, was inspired by a desire to break his own heavy smoking habit. Chinese pharmacist Hon Lik invented the first modern e-cigarette in 2003 after watching his father die of lung cancer. Juul founders Adam Bowen and James Monsees created their revolutionary device with the goal of making traditional cigarettes obsolete.

Despite the stated intentions of e-cigarette innovators, public health officials initially adopted a cautious approach toward vaping. In 2008, for instance, the World Health Organization issued a statement warning individuals and governments that the health claims surrounding e-cigarettes remained unproven. Although WHO officials acknowledged that vaping could potentially play a role in THR, they recommended that e-cigarettes undergo rigorous scientific testing before being approved for widespread use. The WHO warning prompted many countries to ban or impose restrictions on vaping products.

Although the Tobacco Control Act of 2009 did not initially apply to e-cigarettes, which had only recently been introduced in the United States at that time, it included a provision allowing the FDA to deem other products containing nicotine to be tobacco products—and thus subject to restrictions intended to promote public health. As the FDA considered extending its regulatory authority to include e-cigarettes, supporters and opponents engaged in a heated debate about the benefits and risks of vaping. Vaping advocates urged the FDA to preserve access to e-cigarettes for adult smokers of combustible cigarettes, arguing that vaping offered a safer alternative that had the potential to save lives. Vaping opponents, on the other hand, expressed concerns about e-cigarettes' unproven safety record and potential to introduce young people to nicotine. They demanded that the FDA enact strict regulations on e-cigarette manufacturing, advertising, and sales to protect consumers from nicotine addiction and possible health risks.

Both sides cited studies to support their point of view and attacked studies that reached opposite conclusions. Some pro-vaping advocates accused public health officials of exaggerating the health risks of e-cigarettes to protect the interests of big tobacco and pharmaceutical companies, which donated lots of money to fund government research and support political campaigns. "Many of the people who are being paid to conduct the science have been knowingly and intentionally manipulating their results, omitting results, selectively cherry picking and basically misrepresenting their own findings because they're getting federal funding," said THR proponent William Godshall (Gross 2017). Tobacco-control groups countered by claiming that vaping enthusiasts dismissed the potential health risks of e-cigarettes without examining the evidence.

In 2016, the FDA issued its long-awaited "deeming" regulations for vaping products. The rules required e-cigarette manufacturers to provide lists of ingredients, place nicotine warning labels on packaging, and halt the distribution of free samples. The FDA also established a federal minimum age of 18 for the purchase of vaping products. The most controversial provision required e-cigarette manufacturers to submit premarket tobacco applications by August 2018 to receive FDA approval and remain on the market. Critics claimed that complying with the premarket approval requirement would be so complex, expensive, and time-consuming that it would force most of the small, independent e-cigarette companies out of business. They also noted that the FDA granted an exemption from the requirement to tobacco products that had existed in substantially equivalent form prior to February 2007. Although no vaping products qualified for the exemption, it applied to most cigarettes and other traditional tobacco products. Critics charged that it made no sense to apply stricter regulations to e-cigarettes than to combustible cigarettes, which had proven to be far more hazardous to public health.

In 2017, newly elected president Donald Trump appointed Scott Gottlieb as FDA commissioner. Gottlieb initially expressed support for vaping as a means of tobacco harm reduction, noting that "nicotine delivery exists on a continuum of risk" (Gross 2017). He proposed a comprehensive tobacco-control plan that involved reducing nicotine levels in cigarettes to encourage smokers to quit or migrate to less harmful alternatives, including e-cigarettes. Gottlieb responded to the concerns of e-cigarette manufacturers and vaping advocates by delaying the effective date of the premarket approval requirement for five years, until 2022. Vaping supporters celebrated the change, which allowed popular e-cigarette devices and flavors to remain on the market. Public health groups, on the other hand, expressed outrage about the postponement of federal regulation and demanded swift and immediate action to prevent youth vaping.

Youth Vaping and E-Cigarette Regulation

Youth vaping emerged as a pressing public health issue following the 2015 introduction of the Juul e-cigarette. Within three years, Juul accounted for three-quarters of all e-cigarettes sold in the United States. Critics charged that Juul's remarkable sales growth resulted from the innovative device's popularity among teenagers, who began referring to the practice of vaping as "Juuling." Young people appreciated Juul's sleek, attractive, high-tech design. They also liked its compact size and resemblance to a computer memory stick, which made it easier to conceal from parents and teachers. The availability of Juul pods with sweet flavors—such as mango, fruit, crème, and mint—also held appeal for underage users. Juul's high nicotine content and colorful, social media–driven marketing campaign helped vaping become an indelible aspect of youth culture.

From 2017 to 2018, vaping rates increased by 78 percent among high-school students and 48 percent among middle-school students (Cullen et al. 2018). Antismoking advocates worried that the strong appeal of vaping products to young people threatened to reverse decades of gains in tobacco control. In September 2018, Gottlieb declared youth vaping an "epidemic" and threatened to take aggressive steps to prevent e-cigarette use by minors—even if that meant restricting adults' access to the full range of vaping devices and flavors. "The FDA won't tolerate a whole generation of young people becoming addicted to nicotine as a tradeoff for enabling adults to have unfettered access to these same products," he stated. "It's now clear to me that, in closing the on-ramp to kids, we're going to have to narrow the off-ramp for adults who want to migrate off combustible tobacco and onto e-cigs" (Gottlieb 2018).

The FDA announced several changes in its approach to tobacco regulation in light of the youth vaping epidemic. The agency launched educational programs to inform students and parents about the risks of nicotine addiction, stepped up enforcement of laws prohibiting e-cigarette sales to minors, and cracked down on deceptive marketing of vaping products in kid-friendly packaging. Gottlieb gave the leading e-cigarette manufacturers 60 days to develop plans to prevent minors from obtaining their products. If these measures proved ineffective, he threatened to take drastic action, such as prohibiting the sale of flavored e-liquids or requiring e-cigarette manufacturers to submit premarket tobacco approval applications immediately, which would effectively take most vaping products off the market.

In December 2018, Juul's founders announced the sale of a 35 percent stake in their company to Altria (formerly Philip Morris), the producer of

Marlboro cigarettes. Eleven Democratic U.S. senators voiced their disapproval of the deal in a letter, saying, "By accepting $12.8 billion from Altria—a tobacco giant with such a disturbing record of deceptive marketing to hook children onto cigarettes—JUUL has lost what little remaining credibility the company had when it claimed to care about the public health" (Crook 2019). Vaping supporters portray the e-cigarette industry as comprised of small, independent businesses seeking to disrupt cigarette smoking. Yet opponents assert that e-cigarette manufacturing is increasingly dominated by the same powerful tobacco companies that long denied and concealed the dangers of smoking.

Antismoking groups draw many parallels between the business strategies appearing in the unregulated vaping industry and those once used by the tobacco industry. They accuse e-cigarette producers of using deceptive marketing tactics to target children, for instance, as the tobacco industry did prior to federal regulation. They also assert that e-cigarette makers manipulate nicotine levels and delivery systems to maximize their addictive capacity, thus ensuring repeat customers. Critics argue that the vaping industry promotes confusion and skepticism about scientific evidence and attempts to discredit independent studies associating e-cigarettes with harmful health effects. Finally, they point out that pro-vaping groups partner with organizations that have traditionally supported the tobacco industry, such as the Competitive Enterprise Institute and Americans for Tax Reform, to influence policy and delay regulation.

In March 2019, as wrangling over federal regulation of e-cigarettes continued, Gottlieb surprised many observers by announcing his resignation as FDA commissioner. People on both sides of the vaping debate waited anxiously to see whether Gottlieb's successor would continue to advance his policies or proceed in an entirely new direction. In the meantime, the future of vaping swirls in a cloud of controversy.

Further Reading

American Lung Association. 2019. "Smokefree Air Laws." March 8, 2019. https://www.lung.org/our-initiatives/tobacco/smokefree-environments/smokefree-air-laws.html.

Blaha, Michael J. 2019. "Five Things You Need to Know about Vaping." Johns Hopkins Medicine. https://www.hopkinsmedicine.org/health/healthy_heart/know_your_risks/5-truths-you-need-to-know-about-vaping.

CDC. 2018. "Cigarette Smoking among U.S. Adults Lowest Ever Recorded." U.S. Centers for Disease Control and Prevention, November 8, 2018. https://www.cdc.gov/media/releases/2018/p1108-cigarette-smoking-adults.html.

Crook, Jordan. 2019. "Democratic Senators Question Juul about Its Altria Deal." Tech Crunch, April 8, 2019. https://techcrunch.com/2019/04/08/demo cratic-senators-question-juul-about-its-altria-deal/.

Cullen, Karen A., Bridget K. Ambrose, Andrea S. Gentzke, Benjamin J. Apelberg, Ahmed Jamal, and Brian A. King. 2018. "Notes from the Field: Use of Electronic Cigarettes and Any Tobacco Product among Middle and High School Students—United States, 2011–2018." *Morbidity and Mortality Weekly Report* 67 (45): 1276–1277, November 16, 2018. http://dx.doi.org /10.15585/mmwr.mm6745a5.

Fleck, Fiona. 2014. "Countries Vindicate Cautious Stance on E-Cigarettes." *Bulletin of the World Health Organization* 92 (12): 856, December 2014. https:// www.who.int/bulletin/volumes/92/12/14-031214/en/.

Gottlieb, Scott. 2018. "Statement on New Steps to Address Epidemic of Youth E-Cigarette Use." U.S. Food and Drug Administration, September 12, 2018. https://www.fda.gov/NewsEvents/Newsroom/PressAnnouncements /ucm620185.htm.

Gross, Liza. 2017. "Smoke Screen: Big Vape Is Copying Big Tobacco's Playbook." The Verge, November 16, 2017. https://www.theverge.com/2017/11/16/166 58358/vape-lobby-vaping-health-risks-nicotine-big-tobacco-marketing.

Komaroff, Anthony. 2014. "Surgeon General's 1964 Report: Making Smoking History." Harvard Health Publishing, January 10, 2014. https://www .health.harvard.edu/blog/surgeon-generals-1964-report-making-smo king-history-201401106970.

Swartzberg, John. 2018. "Why Tobacco Companies Love E-Cigs." Berkeley Wellness, June 11, 2018. http://www.berkeleywellness.com/self-care/over -counter-products/article/why-tobacco-companies-love-e-cigarettes.

Tolentino, Jia. 2018. "The Promise of Vaping and the Rise of Juul." *New Yorker,* May 14, 2018. https://www.newyorker.com/magazine/2018/05/14/the -promise-of-vaping-and-the-rise-of-juul.

Truth Initiative. 2018. "What You Need to Know to Quit Smoking." November 7, 2018. https://truthinitiative.org/news/what-you-need-know-quit-smoking.

U.S. Department of Health and Human Services. 2018. "The Health Consequences of Smoking—50 Years of Progress: A Report of the Surgeon General." SurgeonGeneral.gov.   https://www.surgeongeneral.gov/library/reports/50 -years-of-progress/fact-sheet.html.

CHAPTER TWO

Landmark Events

This chapter explores important milestones and events in vaping and tobacco use in the United States. It covers the key investigations, lawsuits, legislation, and antismoking campaigns that revealed the deceptive practices of the tobacco industry and raised public awareness of the health risks of cigarette smoking. It also traces the development of electronic cigarettes and charts the phenomenal growth of vaping. Finally, it examines the polarized national debate between vaping supporters, who embrace e-cigarettes as a potentially lifesaving alternative for adult smokers, and tobacco-control advocates, who view vaping as a major health threat for American teenagers.

Invention of the Electronic Cigarette (1963)

Cigarette smoking reached its peak in the United States in 1963, when Americans consumed a record 523 billion cigarettes (White 2018). That same year, inventor Herbert A. Gilbert applied for a patent on a device he called the "smokeless non-tobacco cigarette." Although he never managed to sell the device commercially, Gilbert views his invention as a direct ancestor of the modern e-cigarette. "There is no electric cigarette today, that I have seen, that does not follow the basic road map set forth in my original patent. If you remove any part shown in my original patent from their electric cigarette it will not function," he stated. "Timing can be everything, and I was ahead of my time" (Dunworth 2013). Gilbert's invention predated efforts by the big tobacco companies to create reduced-harm cigarettes and influenced the design of vaping products developed four decades later.

Eliminating Combustion from Smoking

At the time he developed the concept for a smokeless cigarette, Gilbert was a 32-year-old Korean War veteran working in his family's scrap-metal business in the Pittsburgh suburb of Beaver Falls, Pennsylvania. The idea came to him when he saw a neighbor burning leaves and yard waste outdoors, sending foul-smelling smoke into the air. He contrasted that smell with the pleasant aroma of bread baking—rather than burning—in his aunt's bakery. As a longtime smoker of two packs of cigarettes per day, Gilbert regularly inhaled smoke into his lungs. He wondered if it might be possible to replicate the sensation of smoking without producing smoke. "The problem could not occur if there was no combustion. Eureka! I had to find a way to put out the fire," he recalled. "At this point I happened to remember how tea is brewed. That solved the problem. Using logic, I had to find a way to replace burning tobacco and paper with heated, moist, flavored air" (Dunworth 2013).

Gilbert's invention, dubbed the Smokeless, featured a long aluminum cylinder with a silver mouthpiece shaped like a cigarette tip. The cylinder contained a replaceable cartridge filled with flavored liquid. As the user drew air into the cylinder, a battery-powered bulb heated the air. The warm air then passed through the flavored liquid to create a moist vapor, which users inhaled through the mouthpiece into their lungs. Gilbert envisioned the device helping smokers quit by providing the tactile sensations associated with cigarettes without generating smoke from combustion. He also claimed that inhaling vapor with such flavors as cinnamon, mint, and rum could promote weight loss by allowing dieters to "smoke their favorite food" (White 2018). Gilbert also foresaw the device being used to treat lung ailments and to deliver medications in a painless manner.

Unlike modern-day e-cigarettes, Gilbert's device was not intended to deliver nicotine, so he did not attempt to make cartridges containing the chemical stimulant found in tobacco. In addition, the clunky, low-capacity, single-use batteries available in 1963 differed significantly from the powerful, lightweight, rechargeable batteries found in modern vapes. The basic appearance and function of the device resembled e-cigarettes, however, and Gilbert's patent application featured all of the main components included in vapes.

The Smokeless Cigarette Disappears

After Gilbert received a U.S. patent for his smokeless non-tobacco cigarette in 1965, he built prototypes and attempted to sell the manufacturing rights to tobacco companies as well as pharmaceutical firms. The concept attracted little interest, however, and he never found a company willing to mass-produce the device for commercial sale. Gilbert remained convinced that the idea had merit, but he eventually gave up trying to market his invention. He figured that someone else would develop the product when his patent expired in 17 years.

In reality, it took 40 years and many false starts before e-cigarettes finally gained worldwide popularity. While some inventors developed their vaping technologies independently, many others cited Gilbert's 1965 patent as the inspiration for various elements of their designs. In the meantime, Gilbert retired and moved to Florida, where he observed the vaping phenomenon with great interest. Although he never made any money from what many consider to be the world's first e-cigarette, Gilbert expressed pride that his invention helped people quit smoking cigarettes. "The only substantial thing I received was the satisfaction of saving millions of lives," he said (White 2018).

Further Reading

Baker, Phyllis. 2018. "The Debt Owed: A Brief History of Vaping Technology." TechnoFAQ, March 30, 2018. https://technofaq.org/posts/2018/03/the -debt-owed-a-brief-history-of-vaping-technology/.

Dunworth, James. 2012. "The History of the Electronic Cigarette: It Goes Back Further Than You Think. . . ." E-Cigarette Direct Ashtray Blog, May 3, 2012. https://www.ecigarettedirect.co.uk/ashtray-blog/2012/05/history -electronic-cigarette.html.

Dunworth, James. 2013. "An Interview with the Inventor of the Electronic Cigarette, Herbert A. Gilbert." E-Cigarette Direct Ashtray Blog, October 2, 2013. https://www.ecigarettedirect.co.uk/ashtray-blog/2013/10/interview -inventor-e-cigarette-herbert-a-gilbert.html.

White, April. 2018. "Plans for the First E-Cigarette Went Up in Smoke 50 Years Ago." *Smithsonian,* December 2018. https://www.smithsonianmag.com /innovation/plans-for-first-e-cigarette-went-up-in-smoke-50-years-ago -180970730/.

The Surgeon General's Report on Smoking and Health (1964)

Although researchers uncovered evidence of a link between cigarette smoking and lung cancer as early as the 1930s, few Americans understood or worried about the potential health risks. Many people considered smoking hip, fashionable, and an expression of personal freedom. The big tobacco companies reinforced this view in advertisements featuring the rugged Marlboro Man or the liberated Virginia Slims woman. While denying that smoking caused cancer, the cigarette makers also introduced new product innovations that were purported to be safe, such as low-tar, ultra-light, and filtered cigarettes.

Public perceptions changed dramatically in 1964, when U.S. Surgeon General Luther L. Terry (1911–1985) released a bombshell report that eliminated all doubt about the health risks associated with cigarette smoking. On the 50th anniversary of its release, the *Oncology Journal* described *Smoking and Health: Report of the Advisory Committee of the Surgeon General of the Public Health Service* as "one of the most important and most widely quoted documents in the annals of medicine" (Blum 2014). Its publication launched a decades-long battle by lawmakers and public health organizations to reduce U.S. cigarette-smoking rates and hold the tobacco industry accountable for its deceptive practices. The exposure of smoking-related disease risks also led to the development of new nicotine-delivery methods to promote tobacco harm reduction and smoking cessation, including electronic cigarettes.

Formation of the Advisory Committee

As the popularity of cigarettes grew in the early twentieth century, evidence of the health-related dangers of smoking mounted. Dr. Alton Ochsner conducted pioneering research on the subject in the 1930s, after noticing an epidemic of previously rare lung cancers among American servicemen who took up smoking during World War I (1914–1918). Similarly, the British epidemiologist Sir Richard Doll (1912–2005) performed extensive studies to determine the cause of a rapid increase in lung cancer in England following World War II (1939–1945). He found a causal link between smoking and several lung diseases, including bronchitis and emphysema as well as cancer. Yet fellow physicians—the majority of whom were smokers—largely ignored or ridiculed the results of such research. Tobacco companies routinely handed out free samples at medical conferences, and the *Journal of the American Medical Association* (*JAMA*) featured cigarette advertisements until 1954.

The U.S. Public Health Service formally adopted a position recognizing the causal relationship between smoking and lung cancer in 1957. England's Royal College of Physicians followed five years later with a report that also depicted smoking as a contributing factor in cardiovascular disease. Although these reports did not receive much public attention, they did convince a coalition of private health organizations to ask President John F. Kennedy to convene a national commission to find "a solution to this health problem that would interfere least with the freedom of industry or the happiness of individuals" (National Institutes of Health 2018). On June 7, 1962, newly appointed Surgeon General Terry announced plans to form a committee of experts to review the available scientific research on smoking and health.

After soliciting nominations from voluntary medical associations as well as federal agencies—including the American Cancer Society, the American Heart Association, the National Tuberculosis Association, the American Public Health Association, the American Medical Association, the U.S. Food and Drug Administration, the Federal Trade Commission, and the Tobacco Institute—Terry selected ten committee members from various medical disciplines whom he believed would approach the question impartially. Beginning in November 1962, the committee spent the next year reviewing more than 7,000 scientific papers at the National Library of Medicine in Bethesda, Maryland. The advisory committee presented its conclusions in a 386-page report that described smoking as "a health hazard of sufficient importance to warrant appropriate remedial action" by the federal government (Blum 2014).

The Report and Its Impact

Mindful of its potential impact, Terry decided to release the report on a Saturday, which would not only limit its effect on the U.S. stock market but also provide maximum exposure in Sunday newspapers and television news programs. He announced the committee's findings in a press conference on January 11, 1964. Terry began by acknowledging that "few medical questions have stirred such public interest or created more scientific debate than the tobacco-health controversy" (Blum 2014). He went on to provide details from the *Smoking and Health* report about the myriad negative health consequences associated with cigarette smoking. The committee found that smokers faced a 70 percent increase in age-adjusted mortality over nonsmokers, for instance, as well as a risk of developing lung cancer 10 to 20 times higher than nonsmokers. The report also declared smoking to be the primary cause of chronic bronchitis and found a strong correlation between smoking and the incidence of emphysema, heart disease, and newborns with low birthweight.

The report generated some controversy by characterizing smoking as a habit rather than an addiction. Although later studies suggested that nicotine carries a strong potential for physical addiction, many people continued to view smoking as a psychological habit that individuals should be capable of breaking. The federal government weighed in on the question again in 1988, when Surgeon General C. Everett Koop (1916–2013) reversed the 1964 findings and redefined tobacco use as an addiction. He asserted that nicotine met all of the standard criteria for addictive drugs, including mood-altering effects, compulsive use despite adverse consequences, persistent cravings or withdrawal symptoms during abstinence, and frequent relapses after quitting. The tobacco industry disputed the change, however, and continued to portray smoking as a personal choice.

The health claims presented in the 1964 report significantly affected Americans' attitudes about cigarette smoking. Terry recalled that the report "hit the country like a bombshell. It was front page news and a lead story on every radio and television station in the United States and many abroad" (National Institutes of Health 2018). A Gallup poll indicated that the percentage of Americans who believed that smoking caused lung cancer increased from 44 percent in 1958 to 78 percent in 1968 (National Institutes of Health 2018). Millions of people responded to the Surgeon General's warning by quitting smoking, contributing to a decrease in the percentage of Americans who smoked from 42 percent in 1964 to 18 percent in 2014 (Komaroff 2014). According to the *Journal of the American Medical Association*, this decrease prevented 8 million premature deaths over the next 50 years (Holford, Meza, and Warner 2014).

Although the report did not specify actions for the government to take to limit the effects of tobacco use on public health, Congress passed several new laws over the next few years aimed at discouraging cigarette smoking. The Federal Cigarette Labeling and Advertising Act of 1965, for instance, required tobacco companies to place a health warning label on cigarette packages. The Public Health Cigarette Smoking Act of 1969 banned cigarette advertising from American radio and television broadcasts. The Public Health Service also established the National Clearinghouse for Smoking and Health to publicize new research findings about the health impacts of smoking and promote messages and programs aimed at reducing tobacco use. As part of the national antismoking campaign, the Surgeon General and the Office on Smoking and Health in the U.S. Centers for Disease Control and Prevention also produced dozens of additional reports outlining the health risks associated with cigarette smoking.

Further Reading

Blum, Alan. 2014. "Blowing Smoke: The Lost Legacy of the 1964 Surgeon General's Report on Smoking and Health." *Oncology Journal* 28 (5): May 15, 2014. http://www.cancernetwork.com/oncology-journal/blowing-smoke -lost-legacy-1964-surgeon-generals-report-smoking-and-health.

Holford, Theodore R., Rafael Meza, and Kenneth E. Warner. 2014. "Tobacco Control and the Reduction in Smoking-Related Premature Deaths in the United States, 1964–2012." *Journal of the American Medical Association* 311 (2): 164–171, January 8, 2014.

Komaroff, Anthony. 2014. "Surgeon General's 1964 Report: Making Smoking History." Harvard Health Publishing, January 10, 2014. https://www.health.harvard.edu/blog/surgeon-generals-1964-report-making-smoking-history-201401106970.

National Institutes of Health. 2018. "The Reports of the Surgeon General: The 1964 Report on Smoking and Health." U.S. National Library of Medicine. https://profiles.nlm.nih.gov/ps/retrieve/Narrative/NN/p-nid/60.

U.S. Department of Health and Human Services. 2018. "The Health Consequences of Smoking—50 Years of Progress: A Report of the Surgeon General." SurgeonGeneral.gov. https://www.surgeongeneral.gov/library/reports/50-years-of-progress/fact-sheet.html.

Cigarette Warning Labels and Advertising Bans (1965–1970)

Following the release of the Surgeon General's 1964 *Smoking and Health* report, which unequivocally established a link between cigarette smoking and lung cancer, consumer advocates and public health officials called upon lawmakers to regulate the tobacco industry. Over the next few years, the federal government imposed new restrictions on the marketing of tobacco products, including laws that required health warning labels on cigarette packs and banned cigarette advertisements on radio and television. The tobacco industry, meanwhile, worked to downplay the connection between smoking and respiratory illnesses, block or limit warning labels, and challenge restrictions on advertising. Decades later, as vaping exploded in popularity among American teenagers, critics accused e-cigarette manufacturers of adopting the tobacco industry's marketing tactics and demanded similar restrictions on advertisements for vaping products.

Cigarette Warning Labels

As evidence of the harmful effects of smoking increased, antismoking groups pressured state and federal lawmakers to address the growing threat to public health. Some studies suggested that placing health warning labels on cigarette packages offered a low-cost way to raise consumer awareness and influence purchasing behavior. Several state legislatures floated proposals for warning labels during the 1950s. South Dakota lawmakers, for instance, proposed a bill in 1959 that would have required a skull-and-crossbones symbol to appear prominently on every pack of cigarettes.

Spurred by the outcry that followed the Surgeon General's report, Congress passed the Federal Cigarette Labeling and Advertising Act of 1965. The new law mandated that the message "Caution: Cigarette Smoking May Be Hazardous to Your Health" be printed on the side panel of every cigarette package manufactured after January 1, 1966. To avoid subjecting manufacturers to a confusing jumble of regulations, the law also prohibited any further labeling requirements from being enacted at the federal, state, or local levels.

The tobacco lobby initially fought against the warning labels, contending that they violated tobacco companies' free speech rights by forcing them to participate in government-mandated antismoking campaigns. The tobacco industry eventually accepted the warning labels, however, in the belief that the presence of vague health-related messages would not prevent people from smoking. In addition, tobacco insiders pointed out that the law offered companies protection from more onerous state and local packaging requirements.

Public health officials and consumer advocates continued pressing for stronger wording, larger labels, and more prominent placement on cigarette packs. In 1969, Congress responded to these demands by passing the Public Health Cigarette Smoking Act, which changed the health warning labels to read "Warning: The Surgeon General Has Determined That Cigarette Smoking Is Dangerous to Your Health" effective November 1, 1970.

A decade later, a Federal Trade Commission (FTC) report concluded that the existing warning labels had not been effective in informing consumers about the dangers of smoking or changing their attitudes and behavior. The Comprehensive Smoking Education Act of 1984 mandated four new Surgeon General's warnings—each describing specific health risks—to appear on cigarette packaging and advertising material on a quarterly, rotating basis: "Smoking Causes Lung Cancer, Heart Disease, Emphysema, and May Complicate Pregnancy"; "Quitting Smoking Now Greatly Reduces Serious Risks to Your Health"; "Smoking by Pregnant Women May Result in Fetal Injury, Premature Birth, and Low Birth Weight"; and "Cigarette Smoke Contains Carbon Monoxide."

In 1985, the year these warning labels took effect, Iceland became the first nation to require pictorial warning labels—also known as graphic health warning labels (GHWL)—on tobacco products. In Canada and other countries, the images evolved over time to include realistic depictions of the health effects of smoking, such as blackened lungs, decaying teeth, and cancerous growths. Australia and Great Britain passed laws intended to make cigarette packaging as plain and unappealing as possible by removing brand identifiers, restricting fonts, and requiring the use of a muddy brown-green color that reminded consumers of "death and filth" (Blakemore 2016). Critics argue that the United States has fallen behind such international antismoking efforts. Although the U.S. Food and Drug Administration (FDA) proposed a rule requiring GHWL in 2010, the tobacco industry mounted a legal challenge that prevented its implementation.

TV and Radio Advertising Ban

Concern about the Surgeon General's report also led antismoking groups to call for restrictions on the marketing of cigarettes. Tobacco companies ranked among the largest advertisers during the early years of television in the 1950s and 1960s. In fact, Camel cigarettes sponsored the first regular TV news broadcast, NBC's *Camel News Caravan*. As the harmful health effects of smoking became clear, public health officials and consumers worried about the impact of unregulated cigarette advertising on impressionable children. Some critics demanded a federal ban on tobacco advertisements on radio and television.

In 1967, the Federal Communications Commission (FCC) took steps to counteract the influence of cigarette advertising by providing airtime for antismoking messages. FCC officials applied a policy known as the fairness doctrine, which required TV stations to broadcast opposing views on controversial subjects, to ensure that viewers saw one antismoking public-service announcement for every three cigarette commercials. As these anti-tobacco messages raised public awareness of the health risks associated with cigarettes, the number of smokers began to decline.

By 1969, however, tobacco accounted for more commercial airtime than any other product (Glass 2018), and FCC Chairman Rosel Hyde threatened to ban all cigarette advertisements from TV and radio broadcasts. Although the tobacco lobby initially fought the proposed ban, industry representatives realized that removing cigarette commercials from the airwaves would put an end to the antismoking public-service announcements as well as make funds available for other types of advertising. Congress stepped in to pass the Public Health Cigarette Smoking Act, which President Richard Nixon signed into law on April 1, 1970. The act included a ban on radio and television advertising of tobacco products (with the exception of smokeless tobacco products) that took effect on January 2, 1971.

With the broadcast advertising ban in place, the tobacco companies shifted their marketing strategies to emphasize magazines, newspapers, billboards, and mass transit. Expenditures for cigarette advertisements in national magazines grew by 131 percent in the year after the ban took effect. Some critics claimed that the influx of advertising dollars from cigarette manufacturers influenced the content of print media. One study that compared the coverage of smoking-related health issues in leading magazines from the decade prior to the ban to the decade following it found that the coverage decreased by 65 percent (Warner and Goldenhar 1989).

Additional tobacco advertising restrictions were put in place in 1998, following the Master Settlement Agreement that resolved state litigation against the major U.S. tobacco companies. Under the agreement, cigarette manufacturers agreed to stop advertising on billboards and public transportation, end sponsorship of concerts and sporting events, and cease any marketing practices that targeted people under age 18. The Family Smoking Prevention and Tobacco Control Act of 2009 also barred cigarette manufacturers from placing their logos on hats, T-shirts, or other apparel. Since that time, according to the antismoking advocacy organization Truth Initiative, the leading tobacco companies have spent nearly all of their estimated $8.5 billion annual cigarette advertising budget on point-of-sale marketing, such as product displays at supermarkets, pharmacies, convenience stores, and gas stations (Truth Initiative 2017).

Further Reading

Blakemore, Erin. 2016. "The World's 'Ugliest' Color Could Help People Quit Smoking." *Smithsonian*, June 9, 2016. https://www.smithsonianmag.com/smart-news/worlds-ugliest-color-could-help-people-quit-smoking-180959364/#hzGyub3CDbXjPLUa.99.

Brumage, Jody. 2017. "The Public Health Cigarette Smoking Act of 1970." Robert C. Byrd Center, July 25, 2017. https://www.byrdcenter.org/byrd-center-blog/the-public-health-cigarette-smoking-act-of-1970.

Centers for Disease Control and Prevention. 2000. "Smoking and Tobacco Use: Warning Labels." https://www.cdc.gov/tobacco/data_statistics/sgr/2000/highlights/labels/index.htm.

Eschner, Kat. 2017. "People Have Tried to Make U.S. Cigarette Warning Labels More Graphic for Decades." *Smithsonian*, January 11, 2017. https://www.smithsonianmag.com/smart-news/cigarette-warning-labels-more-graphic-180961721/#QeiWGOrC7yfSQLjp.99.

Glass, Andrew. 2018. "Congress Bans Airing Cigarette Ads, April 1, 1970." Politico, April 1, 2018. https://www.politico.com/story/2018/04/01/congress-bans-airing-cigarette-ads-april-1-1970-489882.

Truth Initiative. 2017. "What Do Tobacco Advertising Restrictions Look Like Today?" February 6, 2017. https://truthinitiative.org/news/what-do-tobacco -advertising-restrictions-look-today.

Warner, K. E., and L. M. Goldenhar. 1989. "The Cigarette Advertising Broadcast Ban and Magazine Coverage of Smoking and Health." *Journal of Public Health Policy* 10 (1): 32–42, Spring 1989. https://www.ncbi.nlm.nih.gov /pubmed/2715337.

Development of the First Commercial Vape (1979)

During the 1970s, as growing concerns about the health risks of smoking prompted increased federal regulation of tobacco products, scientists and inventors continued seeking safer alternatives to combustible cigarettes. Some of these early efforts influenced the later development of vaping products. The first known use of the words "vaping" and "vaper" occurred in 1979, more than three decades prior to the introduction of modern e-cigarettes. Dr. Norman Jacobson included the terms in a presentation to colleagues outlining the results of his medical research on non-combustible cigarettes (NCCs). "To simplify description, we will hereafter refer to nicotine vapor inhalation through an NCC as vaping and people who inhale nicotine vapor as vapers," he stated (Jacobson 1979). Although the non-combustible cigarettes Jacobson tested were not electronic, they were among the first commercially available vapes.

An Alternative Method for Nicotine Delivery

Although inventor Herbert A. Gilbert received a U.S. patent for a smokeless electronic cigarette in 1965, his device did not deliver nicotine—the chemical stimulant found in tobacco that causes physical dependency. NCCs, in contrast, were developed specifically to deliver nicotine to users' lungs without smoke. The concept originated with one of Jacobson's patients, Phil Ray, a brilliant computer scientist who helped invent the microprocessor chip and worked on the Apollo space program. As a heavy smoker, Ray understood the health risks associated with cigarettes, yet he had trouble quitting because he was addicted to nicotine. While visiting with his physician, Ray "conceptualized the notion of inhaling the vapor of pure nicotine, the premise and basis for the e-cigarette," Jacobson recalled (Dunworth 2014).

Ray and Jacobson came up with a low-tech design for a plastic tube that looked like a cigarette. Inside the tube, they placed a cartridge containing filter paper soaked in liquid nicotine. When users inhaled through the tube, they received a dose of nicotine. Since the process did not involve combustion or create smoke, the men decided to use the term "vaping" in place of "smoking." They viewed vaping as a healthier way for smokers to ingest nicotine. "If nicotine is truly addicting and if tar, carbon monoxide, and other byproducts of smoking are injurious to health, then obviously, it would be beneficial to develop a cigarette which supplies nicotine, but eliminates the other toxic ingredients," Jacobson explained (Jacobson 1979).

Jacobson recruited other health professionals to help him study the effectiveness of NCCs. They asked six subjects to smoke cigarettes exclusively for four days, and then to vape exclusively for four more days. They tested the subjects daily to measure the level of carbon monoxide in their bloodstream and the level of cotinine (the main metabolite of nicotine) in their urine. The results showed that vaping delivered similar amounts of nicotine as smoking but lowered carbon monoxide to levels similar to those of nonsmokers. In addition, most subjects found vaping satisfying enough that they smoked less.

Bringing NCCs to the Market

Convinced that they had a promising new product idea, Jacobson and Ray formed a company, American Tobacco Products Inc., to produce and sell NCCs. They named their nicotine-delivery system the Favor and advertised its potential health benefits with the slogan "Do Yourself a Favor." Since the Favor did not produce smoke, they marketed it as an option for people to use in places that prohibited cigarette smoking, such as in the workplace or on commercial airlines. They also promoted it as a more satisfying and effective smoking-cessation tool than nicotine tablets, gum, injections, or aerosol sprays.

During the early 1980s, the Favor was sold in grocery chains throughout the western United States. Before long, however, Jacobson and Ray ran into technical and legal issues that forced them to withdraw the product from the market. One problem involved the short shelf life of the Favor. Since pure nicotine degrades rapidly into cotinine, which has a bitter taste and lacks the stimulant properties of nicotine, the product often went bad before it could be sold. In addition, the U.S. Food and Drug Administration ruled that the nicotine-delivery system constituted a "new drug" that could not be sold without federal approval. Rather than submitting the product for an expensive and drawn-out approval process, Jacobson and Ray sold the technology to Upjohn in Sweden and closed their company.

Although Ray died in 1987, Jacobson witnessed the development of modern e-cigarettes, which resolved many of the technical issues that had affected the Favor. "Frankly the electronic device is a superior device because the nicotine is encapsulated and so it is protected from the vaporizing until it's heated, which is a very clever idea," he said (Dunworth 2014). He also saw vaping become a global phenomenon, using the terminology he introduced three decades earlier.

Further Reading

Baker, Phyllis. 2018. "The Debt Owed: A Brief History of Vaping Technology." TechnoFAQ, March 30, 2018. https://technofaq.org/posts/2018/03/the-debt-owed-a-brief-history-of-vaping-technology/.

Dunworth, James. 2012. "The History of the Electronic Cigarette: It Goes Back Further Than You Think. . . ." E-Cigarette Direct Ashtray Blog, May 3, 2012. https://www.ecigarettedirect.co.uk/ashtray-blog/2012/05/history-electronic-cigarette.html.

Dunworth, James. 2014. "Vaping 1970s Style: An Interview with One of the Pioneers." E-Cigarette Direct Ashtray Blog, June 23, 2014. https://www.ecigarettedirect.co.uk/ashtray-blog/2014/06/favor-cigarette-interview-dr-norman-jacobson.html.

Jacobson, Norman L. 1979. "Non-Combustible Cigarette: Alternative Method of Nicotine Delivery." Paper presented to the American College of Chest Physicians. UCSF Library, Truth Tobacco Industry Documents. https://www.industrydocumentslibrary.ucsf.edu/tobacco/docs/#id=kswx0210.

Tobacco Industry Litigation and Settlements (1998–2006)

From the time that the American people became aware of the harmful health effects associated with cigarette smoking, various individuals and groups attempted to hold the tobacco industry legally responsible for selling a dangerous product. They finally succeeded during the late 1990s and early 2000s, when investigations, lawsuits, and documents provided by whistleblowers revealed decades of deception and fraud by the leading cigarette manufacturers. These revelations severely damaged the big tobacco companies' public image and credibility, which raised questions about their involvement in the vaping industry and fueled doubts about their commitment to tobacco harm reduction.

The Tobacco Industry Avoids Liability

Beginning in 1954, smokers and their families filed hundreds of lawsuits against cigarette manufacturers. They claimed the tobacco companies misrepresented their products as safe and acted with negligence by knowingly selling products that caused addiction and disease. The plaintiffs sought monetary damages to reimburse medical expenses, lost wages, and pain and suffering. Attorneys for the tobacco companies managed to get most of the cases dismissed, however, and won the few that went to trial. Their early strategy involved denying that cigarette smoking caused disease, questioning the credibility of the medical evidence, and rejecting the idea that manufacturers had a duty to warn consumers.

After the 1964 Surgeon General's report revealed an explicit link between smoking and lung cancer, the federal government required warning labels to be placed on cigarette packages. The tobacco companies then adopted a new defense against personal injury lawsuits, claiming that they were immune from liability because consumers had been informed about the health risks of smoking. Industry lawyers argued that individual smokers knowingly accepted these risks and thus bore legal responsibility for the impact of their decision to smoke. The leading cigarette manufacturers strenuously defended themselves against all litigation, using their wealth and resources to make court battles as expensive and time consuming as possible for the plaintiffs, and prevailed in nearly every case.

The lone exception came in the 1983 case of Rose Cipollone, a New Jersey woman who smoked more than a pack of cigarettes per day from age 16 until her death from lung cancer at 53. Unable to quit smoking, Cipollone switched cigarette brands several times, always choosing filtered or light cigarettes that the manufacturers advertised as healthier alternatives. Her attorney focused on these health claims, arguing that the tobacco companies had committed fraud by misrepresenting dangerous products as healthy in direct contradiction of the government health warnings. In the first significant loss for the tobacco industry, a jury awarded Cipollone's family $400,000 in damages. The verdict was quickly overturned on appeal, however, and the case wound its way through the legal system for nearly a decade before reaching the U.S. Supreme Court in 1992 in *Cipollone v. Liggett Group, Inc.*, 505 U.S. 504. Although the high court's split ruling denied damages to Cipollone's family, it also provided a road map for future litigants, suggesting that they would have a chance of prevailing if they could prove the tobacco industry had hidden or lied about the hazards of smoking.

In the meantime, the U.S. Food and Drug Administration (FDA), under the leadership of Commissioner David A. Kessler (1951–), launched an investigation of the tobacco industry and its impact on public health. Kessler sought to define nicotine as an addictive drug to make tobacco subject to FDA regulation. His investigation uncovered evidence that cigarette manufacturers had intentionally manipulated the levels of nicotine in their products to increase their addictive potential. Kessler also found evidence that the tobacco companies withheld information from investigators, suppressed scientific research findings, and specifically targeted underage youth to create a new generation of smokers to replace those who quit or succumbed to smoking-related illnesses.

The 1994 Tobacco Hearings

Kessler's investigation prompted the U.S. House of Representatives to conduct a series of hearings examining the public health impacts of cigarette smoking and the business practices of the tobacco industry. One of the most notable moments occurred on April 14, 1994, when the heads of the seven largest U.S. tobacco companies appeared before a congressional subcommittee chaired by Representative Henry Waxman (D-CA). During six hours of intensive questioning, all seven tobacco executives denied under oath that nicotine was addictive and insisted that smoking was a personal choice. Although they acknowledged that their companies manipulated the level of nicotine in cigarettes, they claimed that the purpose was to enhance flavor rather than to cause smokers to become hooked.

The spectacle of the congressional hearings, which were broadcast live on cable television, led to public outrage and increased calls for federal regulation of the tobacco industry. It also encouraged several whistleblowers to come forward with industry documents contradicting the tobacco executives' sworn testimony. Merrell Williams Jr. came across incriminatory memos, correspondence, and research results while working as a paralegal for a Kentucky law firm that represented the tobacco giant Brown and Williamson, makers of Kool, Pall Mall, and dozens of other popular cigarette brands. One internal memo—written by Brown and Williamson's vice president and general counsel, Addison Yeaman— proved that the company knew about nicotine's addictive properties as early as 1963. "Nicotine is addictive," Yeaman wrote. "We are, then, in the business of selling nicotine, an addictive drug effective in the release of stress mechanisms" (Chawkins 2013).

Another key informant was Jeffrey Wigand, a former research and development executive for Brown and Williamson who cooperated with Kessler's FDA investigation. Wigand provided insider information showing that the tobacco companies knowingly added toxic chemicals to cigarettes in order to increase the effects of nicotine. In 1996, despite facing threats and legal repercussions, Wigand appeared on the news program

60 Minutes and told a national television audience about the deceptive and dangerous practices he witnessed in the tobacco industry.

The State Cases and the 1998 Master Settlement Agreement

Documents and testimony from whistleblowers helped a group of state attorneys general build a case against the tobacco companies. Mike Moore, attorney general for Mississippi from 1988 to 2004, filed the first state lawsuit in May 1994, and most other states quickly followed. The suit contended that the tobacco industry created a public health crisis that forced the states to pay millions of extra dollars through Medicaid and other health care programs to treat smoking-related illnesses. "Things such as lung cancer, heart disease, emphysema, low-birth-weight babies and others, we have to pay," Moore explained. "The state is obligated to pay for those for our citizens that are not covered in other ways, and we feel like they're caused by the tobacco products" (NPR 2013). The attorneys general accused the tobacco companies of using fraudulent and deceptive marketing practices in violation of consumer-protection statutes, as well as engaging in a conspiracy to conceal the health hazards of smoking in violation of antitrust laws. They also asserted that the tobacco companies intentionally targeted children to create new customers and systematically stifled the development of safer cigarettes, including non-combustible products.

The state cases avoided several traps that had sunk the legal claims made by earlier plaintiffs. The tobacco industry had successfully defended itself against lawsuits brought by individual smokers, for instance, by arguing that the plaintiffs had freely chosen to use tobacco products despite the known risks and thus bore personal responsibility for their actions. Since the state governments did not voluntarily accept these risks, however, this reasoning did not apply to the monetary injuries they incurred from treating smoking-related diseases. In addition, the tobacco companies had often used their significant advantages in financial and legal resources to prevail in cases brought by individual smokers. By combining their claims into a large-scale class-action lawsuit, however, the states negated these advantages.

The state cases against the tobacco industry resulted in the largest legal settlements in U.S. history. Beginning in May 1998, four states—Florida, Minnesota, Mississippi, and Texas—reached individual settlements that required the tobacco industry to pay them a total of $40 billion. Six months later, the attorneys general of the other 46 states, the District of Columbia, Puerto Rico, and the Virgin Islands entered into the Master

Settlement Agreement. This agreement required the four tobacco companies that controlled 97 percent of the U.S. cigarette market—Brown and Williamson, Lorillard, Philip Morris, and R. J. Reynolds—to pay the states and territories a minimum of $206 billion over 25 years. In addition to these four major tobacco companies, known as the Original Participating Manufacturers (OPMs), more than 40 smaller firms later joined the settlement.

The monetary settlement included a series of annual payments to compensate the states for health care costs associated with smoking-related illnesses. Some of the money was also earmarked for the establishment of antismoking research initiatives, campaigns, and advocacy groups. In addition to state and local smoking-cessation programs, for example, it funded the creation of the Truth Initiative, a nonprofit tobacco-control organization focused on preventing youth smoking. Under the Master Settlement Agreement, the OPMs also agreed to dissolve industry-funded groups that promoted fraudulent scientific claims or sought to hide the negative health effects of smoking, such as the Center for Indoor Air Research, the Council for Tobacco Research, and the Tobacco Institute. The agreement also prohibited the OPMs from engaging in marketing practices designed to appeal to young people, such as placing cigarette brand names on T-shirts and merchandise or making tobacco products visible in movies and entertainment. Finally, the agreement required the tobacco companies to make 35 million pages of secret, internal documents available to the public. These documents revealed longstanding industry efforts to deceive consumers about the harmful health effects of smoking.

Despite the massive size of the settlement, some critics contend that it did not go far enough in punishing the tobacco companies for decades of wrongdoing. One area of complaint focuses on the fact that the agreement gave the tobacco industry immunity from future state and federal lawsuits. "With unprecedented future legal protection granted by the state [attorneys general] in exchange for money, it appears that the tobacco industry has emerged from the state lawsuits even more powerful," said antismoking advocate William Godshall (Godshall 1999). As the Master Settlement Agreement neared its 20th anniversary, critics also noted that state governments spent less than 3 percent of their annual tobacco settlement funds—or $721 million of the $27 billion collected in 2018—on tobacco-control programs and cancer research, compared to the 14 percent recommended by the Centers for Disease Control and Prevention (Phend 2018).

Some antismoking advocates argue that the states missed a valuable opportunity to reduce tobacco use and save money on future health care costs by funding smoking-prevention and -cessation programs. "The reality is that for decades the tobacco industry lied about their addictive and deadly products, hooking kids and adults alike for life," said American Lung Association president Harold Wimmer. "The settlement funds have the potential to serve as a lifeline for the millions of Americans now living with a tobacco-related disease" (Phend 2018). Instead, many states diverted tobacco-settlement payments to their general funds, where they went toward such projects as road repair, tax relief, or literacy programs. In a few cases, states applied the money to projects that benefited the tobacco industry. North Carolina once spent 75 percent of its funds to increase tobacco production, for instance, while South Carolina dedicated 15 percent to subsidize tobacco farmers for the effects of price decreases.

The Federal RICO Case

One year after the Master Settlement Agreement concluded the litigation between the major tobacco companies and the states, the federal government brought its own case against cigarette manufacturers under the Racketeer Influenced and Corrupt Organizations (RICO) Act of 1970, which applied to organized criminal activity by business enterprises. The U.S. Department of Justice (DOJ) accused the tobacco companies of violating RICO laws by conspiring to suppress evidence of the health risks of smoking and the addictive capacity of nicotine, manipulating the level of nicotine in cigarettes to maintain addiction, misrepresenting light cigarettes as healthier alternatives, and marketing hazardous products to minors. After six years of litigation, U.S. District Court Judge Gladys Kessler ruled in favor of the DOJ on August 17, 2006.

Her 1,500-page decision in *United States v. Philip Morris* outlined the many ways in which the tobacco industry had pursued profits at the expense of public health. "Over the course of more than 50 years, Defendants lied, misrepresented, and deceived the American public, including smokers and the young people they avidly sought as 'replacement smokers,' about the devastating health effects of smoking and environmental tobacco smoke," Judge Kessler wrote. "They suppressed research, they destroyed documents, they manipulated the use of nicotine so as to increase and perpetuate addiction, they distorted the truth about low tar and light cigarettes so as to discourage smokers from quitting, and they abused the legal system to achieve their goal—to make money with little, if any, regard for individual illness and suffering, soaring health costs, or the integrity of the legal system" (American Cancer Society 2018).

The ruling gave the DOJ several options for preventing future violations by the tobacco industry, such as prohibiting certain marketing practices, requiring disclosure of secret documents, and compelling the release of "corrective statements" to inform the public about health issues the cigarette manufacturers had lied about in the past. Following a series of appeals, the corrective statements were finalized and publicized in 2018—nearly two decades after the DOJ initially filed its lawsuit. The statements covered five main areas of tobacco industry deception: the adverse health effects of smoking; the addictiveness of nicotine; the manipulation of nicotine levels in cigarettes; the lack of health benefits conferred by smoking cigarettes labeled "light," "low-tar," "mild," or "natural"; and the adverse health effects of secondhand smoke. Messages on these topics appeared on cigarette packages, on tobacco company websites, and in newspaper and television advertisements. Some examples of specific statements include:

- Smoking kills, on average, 1,200 Americans. Every day.
- More people die every year from smoking than from murder, AIDS, suicide, drugs, car crashes, and alcohol, combined.
- Smoking causes heart disease, emphysema, acute myeloid leukemia, and cancer of the mouth, esophagus, larynx, lung, stomach, kidney, bladder, and pancreas.
- Smoking is highly addictive. Nicotine is the addictive drug in tobacco.
- Cigarette companies intentionally designed cigarettes with enough nicotine to create and sustain addiction.
- When you smoke, the nicotine actually changes the brain—that's why quitting is so hard.
- Many smokers switch to low-tar and light cigarettes rather than quitting because they think low-tar and light cigarettes are less harmful. They are not.
- Secondhand smoke kills over 38,000 Americans each year.
- Children exposed to secondhand smoke are at an increased risk for sudden infant death syndrome (SIDS), acute respiratory infections, ear problems, severe asthma, and reduced lung function (American Cancer Society 2018).

Further Reading

American Cancer Society. 2018. "Department of Justice Lawsuit against the Tobacco Industry." Cancer Action Network, November 27, 2018. https://www.fightcancer.org/news/department-justice-lawsuit-against-tobacco-industry.

Blanke, D. Douglas. 2002. "Towards Health with Justice: Litigation and Public Inquiries as Tools for Tobacco Control." World Health Organization. https://www.publichealthlawcenter.org/sites/default/files/resources /who-tobacco-litigation-2002.pdf.

Chawkins, Steve. 2013. "Merrell Williams Jr. Dies at 72; Former Paralegal Fought Big Tobacco." *Los Angeles Times,* November 27, 2013. https://www.latimes .com/local/obituaries/la-me-merrell-williams-20131128-story.html.

Godshall, William T. 1999. "Giving 10 Percent to Gain Eternity." *Tobacco Control* 8: 437–439, December 1, 1999. https://tobaccocontrol.bmj.com/content /8/4/437.

"Inside the Tobacco Deal." 1998. PBS Frontline, May 1998. https://www.pbs.org /wgbh/pages/frontline/shows/settlement/.

NPR Staff. 2013. "15 Years Later, Where Did All the Cigarette Money Go?" NPR, October 13, 2013. https://www.npr.org/2013/10/13/233449505/15-years -later-where-did-all-the-cigarette-money-go.

Phend, Crystal. 2018. "Tobacco Master Settlement at 20 Years." MedPage Today, November 24, 2018. https://www.medpagetoday.com/primarycare/smo king/76496.

"State of Tobacco Control." 2018. American Lung Association. https://www.lung .org/our-initiatives/tobacco/reports-resources/sotc/key-findings/.

Introduction of the Modern E-Cigarette (2003)

After investigations and litigation forced cigarette manufacturers to acknowledge the health risks of smoking, the tobacco industry stepped up its efforts to develop reduced-harm alternatives, including smokeless cigarettes. Independent inventors continued working on the problem as well, and in 2003 a Chinese pharmacist named Hon Lik patented what is widely considered the first modern electronic cigarette. Although American inventor Herbert A. Gilbert patented a similar device in 1965, Hon's version was the first widely marketed device to include all the elements of modern vaping technology. As a heavy smoker who watched his father die of lung cancer, Hon originally built it as a smoking-cessation tool, and he expressed hope that vaping would replace cigarette smoking someday. "It's like a digital camera taking over from the analog camera," he explained. "It needs time" (AFP 2013).

Development of Vaping Technology

After ignoring or suppressing independent efforts to develop non-combustible cigarettes, the leading tobacco companies finally launched their own design programs aimed at reducing the harmful health effects of smoking, and especially those associated with exposure to secondhand smoke. R. J. Reynolds introduced the Eclipse, a "heat-not-burn" cigarette that used a carbon fuel rod in its tip to heat tobacco, releasing flavor and nicotine but limiting smoke. Philip Morris released the Accord, an electronic, puff-activated heating mechanism in a box that worked with specially designed cigarettes to produce less smoke than traditional cigarettes. Brown and Williamson established the secretive Vapotronics Group, a research and development team charged with bringing a smokeless electronic cigarette to market. Some new product design efforts in the 1990s that focused on the inhalation of nicotine, however, faced the threat of FDA regulation as drug-delivery devices.

The breakthrough eventually happened in China, where Hon worked in an agricultural research lab designing new methods for consumers to ingest substances that were popular remedies in Chinese traditional medicine. When his father developed lung cancer, Hon grew determined to quit smoking and began wearing nicotine patches. Although the patches did not curb his craving for nicotine, they occasionally produced vivid dreams. "In the evenings I sometimes forgot to take off my nicotine patch," he recalled, "which gave me nightmares all night" (AFP 2013). In one such dream, Hon felt as if he were drowning in an ocean when the water suddenly vaporized, leaving him floating in a colorful cloud. Hon claimed that this dream inspired him to invent a smokeless cigarette that worked by vaporizing nicotine.

Determined to replicate the experience of smoking cigarettes as closely as possible, Hon looked for a liquid base that could deliver nicotine and flavoring while forming a smokelike vapor. After testing several solutions, he decided upon propylene glycol, a nontoxic food additive that is still used in modern e-liquid or vape juice. Hon's initial patent used high-frequency ultrasound waves to vaporize the liquid. After further testing, however, Hon found that using a battery-powered heating coil, known as an atomizer, produced a more satisfying vapor. The next step involved shrinking the device from the size of a computer console to a size that could easily fit in a user's pocket or purse. The availability of high-capacity, rechargeable lithium ion batteries, such as those found in smartphones, simplified the process of scaling down the device. Although the final design resembled Gilbert's patent, which had long expired, it is unclear whether Hon was aware of the earlier invention.

Vaping's Popularity Inspires Further Innovation

Hon called his electronic cigarette Ruyan, meaning "like smoke" in Chinese, and received a patent in China in 2003. Hon produced and marketed Ruyan through the company he worked for, Golden Dragon Holdings, which later became Ruyan Group and then Dragonite International. When Ruyan first hit the Chinese market in 2004, the product proved to be so popular with consumers that the company had trouble meeting demand. The following year, however, a series of media reports claimed that the e-cigarette was responsible for increases in nicotine addiction and heart attacks. Hon accused China's state-run tobacco industry of planting the negative stories because Ruyan's success threatened its sales revenues. "All tobacco companies disliked our products, especially the large ones, and they have influence over governments," he noted. "It's like how the inventor of a perpetual motion machine would receive pressure from the energy industry" (AFP 2013).

Even as the Ruyan faced pressure within China, Hon's company patented the invention in other countries and began exporting e-cigarettes in 2005. Two years later, the first e-cigarettes hit the U.S. market. As the popularity of vaping spread, competitors sprang up selling variations on Hon's design. In addition, enthusiastic vapers joined online forums to exchange information, debate the pros and cons of different features, and discuss ways to improve and customize the vaping experience. Some hobbyists began tinkering with commercially available e-cigarettes to increase their battery life, improve their performance, or change their appearance. In 2007, for instance, Umer and Tariq Sheikh integrated the atomizer into the e-liquid cartridge to create a cartomizer. Later that year, father-and-son vapers Matt and Ted Rogers created a popular modification, or "mod," known as the Screwdriver by replacing the body of an e-cigarette with the metal housing of an oddly shaped flashlight, making it more attractive and durable. The evolution of the technology continued in 2009 with the introduction of the clearomizer, an all-in-one atomizer coil and e-liquid chamber made out of transparent glass or plastic to enable vapers to monitor and refill the vape juice.

By 2014, vaping had grown into a $5 billion global industry, yet Hon received little compensation or recognition for his contributions. Although he signed a $75 million agreement with Imperial Tobacco, one of Europe's largest tobacco companies, for the rights to the e-cigarette patents he developed for Dragonite, Hon received only a small fraction of the proceeds. Industry analysts noted that the fast-paced innovation in vaping technology had rendered his components less valuable. In addition, some vaping enthusiasts criticized his decision to partner with a traditional cigarette maker, since he had experienced the harmful health effects of smoking. Hon responded by arguing that Imperial had the marketing strength to introduce more smokers to vaping. "By using the existing distribution channels of the tobacco companies to tobacconists, maybe it is the best way for consumers to access e-cigarettes," he stated (Boseley 2015). Despite the lack of financial rewards, Hon expressed pride in his invention of a device with the potential to help people quit smoking. "Smoking is the most unhealthy thing in people's everyday lives," he noted. "I've made a big contribution to society" (AFP 2013).

Further Reading

AFP. 2013. "China's E-Cigarette Inventor Fights for Financial Rewards." Fox News, October 1, 2013. https://www.foxnews.com/world/chinas-e-cig arette-inventor-fights-for-financial-rewards.

Boseley, Sarah. 2015. "Hon Lik Invented the E-Cigarette to Quit Smoking—But Now He's a Dual User." *Guardian,* June 9, 2015. https://www.theguard ian.com/society/2015/jun/09/hon-lik-e-cigarette-inventor-quit-smoking -dual-user.

Dunworth, James. 2012. "The History of the Electronic Cigarette: It Goes Back Further Than You Think. . . ." E-Cigarette Direct Ashtray Blog, May 3, 2012. https://www.ecigarettedirect.co.uk/ashtray-blog/2012/05/history -electronic-cigarette.html.

"Hon Lik: The Man Who Invented Vaping." 2016. blu, July 7, 2016. https://www .blu.com/en/US/blog/industry-news/hon-lik-man-invented-vaping.html.

Ridley, Matt. 2015. "'Quitting Is Suffering': Hon Lik, Inventor of the E-Cigarette, on Why He Did It." *Spectator,* June 20, 2015. https://www.spectator .co.uk/2015/06/quitting-is-suffering-hon-lik-inventor-of-the-e-cigarette -on-why-he-did-it/.

The World Health Organization Issues a Warning about E-Cigarettes (2008)

Following their invention in 2003, electronic cigarettes quickly spread around the world. Their popularity was largely driven by manufacturers' claims that vaping offered a safer alternative to traditional tobacco products that could also help smokers give up cigarettes. In 2008, the World Health Organization (WHO)—the United Nations (UN) agency that leads the global response to public health issues—issued a statement warning individuals and governments that the health claims surrounding vaping products remained unproven. Although WHO officials acknowledged that vaping could potentially play a role in tobacco harm reduction, they insisted that e-cigarettes should undergo rigorous scientific testing before being approved for widespread use. The WHO warning prompted many countries, including the United States, to impose restrictions on vaping products.

E-Cigarette Makers Claim Health Benefits

Inventor Hon Lik developed the first modern electronic cigarette with a goal of creating a less hazardous method of nicotine delivery that still gave smokers the tactile sensations they associated with combustible cigarettes. Following the successful introduction of his Ruyan e-cigarette in China, Hon began exporting the device in 2005. As e-cigarettes gained popularity around the world, entrepreneurs and hobbyists modified Hon's original design to improve its functionality and appearance. Like the Ruyan, many of the early e-cigarette models were marketed as reduced-harm alternatives that could help people quit smoking cigarettes.

The WHO helps governments develop policies to control tobacco use in order to prevent smoking-related diseases and premature deaths. In 2003, the WHO adopted the Framework Convention on Tobacco Control (FCTC), a landmark treaty that established global standards intended to "protect present and future generations from the devastating health, social, environmental, and economic consequences of tobacco consumption and exposure to tobacco smoke" (WHO FCTC 2003). The convention achieved ratification by 168 countries and took effect in 2005. Due to concerns raised by the tobacco industry about the treaty's potential economic impact, the United States remained a non-party to it.

One provision of the FCTC requires nations to "take effective measures to promote cessation of tobacco use and adequate treatment for tobacco dependence" (WHO FCTC 2003). Research has suggested that nicotine replacement therapy (NRT) can be a valuable tool in smoking-cessation efforts. Nicotine is the chemical stimulant in tobacco products that has been shown to create physical dependency or addiction. NRT involves delivering small doses of nicotine through such methods as skin patches, chewing gum, lozenges, nasal sprays, and inhalers, which are considered less hazardous than inhaling smoke from combustible cigarettes. For some people, NRT reduces cravings and relieves withdrawal symptoms, enabling them to quit smoking successfully. The WHO and the U.S. Food and Drug Administration (FDA) subject NRT products to rigorous scientific testing before approving them for consumer use in smoking-cessation programs.

The WHO Calls for Testing

E-cigarettes appeared on the scene shortly after the FCTC took effect. Some e-cigarette manufacturers marketed their products as healthier forms of nicotine delivery that could help tobacco users alleviate the desire to smoke. A few producers either claimed or implied that their devices met FCTC standards for NRT products. "Manufacturers of this electronic cigarette around the world have included WHO's name or logo, for example, on their website, on package inserts, or on advertisements," said Douglas Bettcher, director of the WHO's Tobacco Free Initiative (CBC News 2008).

As health claims associated with e-cigarettes proliferated online, public health experts grew concerned that millions of people were adopting the new technology before it had been adequately tested. On September 19, 2008, WHO officials issued a formal statement warning individuals and governments that the alleged benefits of vaping remained unproven. "The electronic cigarette is not a proven nicotine replacement therapy," WHO medical expert Ala Alwan declared in a press conference. "WHO has no scientific evidence to confirm the product's safety and efficacy. Its marketers should immediately remove from their websites and other informational materials any suggestion that WHO considers it to be a safe and effective smoking cessation aid" (O'Leary and Laniel 2008).

Although WHO scientists acknowledged the possibility that e-cigarettes might help people quit smoking, they insisted that such claims must be supported by rigorous, peer-reviewed scientific research. "If the marketers of the electronic cigarette want to help smokers quit, then they need to conduct clinical studies and toxicity analyses and operate within the proper regulatory framework," Bettcher stated. "Until they do that, WHO cannot consider the electronic cigarette to be an appropriate nicotine replacement therapy, and it certainly cannot accept false suggestions that it has approved and endorsed the product" (O'Leary and Laniel 2008).

In addition to the lack of scientific testing, WHO officials cited several other concerns about the rapid adoption of e-cigarettes. They noted, for instance, that it was impossible to predict the long-term health effects of vaping. They also warned about the potential for unregulated e-liquid formulations to contain toxic chemicals or lung irritants. WHO medical experts also argued that variations in device performance, nicotine concentration, and user behavior could lead to nicotine poisoning or overdose. Finally, they pointed to evidence suggesting that some people used e-cigarettes as a means of evading smoking bans in public places rather than as a smoking-cessation tool. They asserted that public health agencies should encourage smokers to end their nicotine addictions rather than enabling them to continue administering nicotine in more socially acceptable forms.

E-Cigarettes Are Subject to Bans and Regulations

The WHO warning about e-cigarettes convinced several FCTC signatory nations to ban the devices, including Australia, Brazil, Canada, Hong Kong, Panama, and Saudi Arabia. In the United States, Senator Frank R. Lautenberg (D-NJ)—an outspoken antismoking advocate who wrote the legislation that banned smoking on commercial airline flights—responded by calling on the FDA to prohibit the sale of e-cigarettes until studies confirmed their safety. By early 2009, however, Americans could easily obtain e-cigarettes on the Internet or from shopping-mall kiosks. Several of Lautenberg's colleagues objected to the proposed ban and offered testimonials to the effectiveness of e-cigarettes as smoking-cessation tools. "Before the FDA takes any immediate action, it should put forward scientific evidence that these products are harmful or unsafe," said Senator Cliff Stearns (R-FL) (Yager 2009).

In March 2009, the FDA informed e-cigarette manufacturers that it planned to block shipments of the devices into the United States. Since the agency did not have regulatory authority over tobacco products at that time, officials attempted to define e-cigarettes as drug-delivery systems, which require FDA approval and registration before they can be sold to the public. E-cigarette manufacturers immediately filed a lawsuit challenging FDA jurisdiction and received an injunction to prevent the ban from taking effect. Federal courts later rejected the FDA's bid to regulate e-cigarettes as drug-delivery systems. In June 2009, Congress passed the Family Smoking Prevention and Tobacco Control Act, which granted the FDA authority to regulate the content, manufacture, marketing, and sale of tobacco products. The FDA eventually deemed e-cigarettes to be tobacco products and thus gained jurisdiction to regulate vaping.

In the meantime, the FDA issued a press release in July 2009 that echoed many of the WHO's warnings about e-cigarettes. "The FDA is concerned about the safety of these products and how they are marketed to the public," FDA Commissioner Margaret A. Hamburg stated (FDA Consumer Health Information 2009). The FDA discouraged consumers from using e-cigarettes until the agency undertook a full review of the products' components, ingredients, labeling, and intended use. FDA officials claimed that initial studies had detected the presence of toxic chemicals, such as diethylene glycol, in e-liquids. They also warned that e-cigarettes could be sold without health warnings or age restrictions, while their attractive product designs and appealing flavors made them enticing to children. Public health experts expressed concern that young people who experimented with vaping could develop nicotine addictions and become more likely to try other tobacco products or illegal drugs.

Further Reading

CBC News. 2008. "Electronic Cigarettes No Safe Alternative to Tobacco, WHO Warns." CBC/Radio Canada, September 19, 2008. https://www.cbc.ca /news/technology/electronic-cigarettes-no-safe-alternative-to-tobacco -who-warns-1.732985.

FDA Consumer Health Information. 2009. "FDA Warns of Health Risks Posed by E-Cigarettes." U.S. Food and Drug Administration, July 2009. http:// www.casaa.org/wp-content/uploads/FDA-Press-Release-2009.pdf.

O'Leary, Timothy A., and Stéfanie Laniel. 2008. "Marketers of Electronic Ciga- rettes Should Halt Unproved Therapy Claims." World Health Organiza- tion, September 19, 2008. https://www.who.int/mediacentre/news/rele ases/2008/pr34/en/.

WHO Framework Convention on Tobacco Control. 2003. Geneva: World Health Organization. https://apps.who.int/iris/bitstream/handle/10665/42811 /9241591013.pdf.

Yager, Jordy. 2009. "Senator Lautenberg Wants to Snuff Out Electronic Cigarettes." *The Hill,* March 23, 2009. https://thehill.com/homenews/news/18879-sen -lautenberg-wants-to-snuff-out-electronic-cigarettes.

The Family Smoking Prevention and Tobacco Control Act (2009)

As a popular consumer product that did not fit neatly into the category of food or drug, tobacco largely avoided being subjected to government regulation for decades. Until the 1964 Surgeon General's report revealed the connection between cigarette smoking and lung cancer, the powerful tobacco lobby successfully resisted most federal oversight, and tobacco- control measures were limited to tepid warning labels on cigarette pack- ages and a ban on broadcast advertising. Even as evidence accumulated of the harmful health effects associated with smoking, tobacco executives denied the addictive properties of nicotine and portrayed smoking as a personal choice that individuals had the freedom to make despite the risks.

During the late 1980s and early 1990s, growing concerns about the risks of secondhand smoke led to renewed calls for federal regulation of tobacco products. Many antismoking advocates argued that the U.S. Food and Drug Administration (FDA)—which oversaw the health and safety of food, drugs, medical devices, and cosmetics marketed and sold to Ameri- can consumers—should have authority over the tobacco industry. Under the leadership of Commissioner David A. Kessler, the FDA sought to define nicotine as an addictive drug and cigarettes as drug-delivery devices. Although the U.S. Supreme Court ruled in 2000 that the FDA lacked the jurisdiction to regulate tobacco products, Congress granted the agency the necessary authority through the Family Smoking Prevention and Tobacco Control Act of 2009. Although the law did not initially apply to e-cigarettes, which had only recently become available in the United States, vaping advocates worried that its provisions might harm the emerging industry. In 2016, the FDA used the act's "deeming" provision to define e-cigarettes as tobacco products and gain regulatory authority over the vaping industry.

The Supreme Court Denies FDA Jurisdiction over Tobacco

The FDA grew out of the wide-reaching reforms of the Progressive Era, when Congress passed a flurry of legislation intended to protect American consumers from unsafe products and unsanitary manufacturing processes. The agency was established under the Pure Food and Drug Act of 1906 to enforce standards for the composition, manufacturing, marketing, and sale of food products, pharmaceutical drugs, and medical devices. It gained additional regulatory powers under the Food, Drug, and Cosmetic Act of 1938, including the authority to require manufacturers to prove the safety and efficacy of drugs before marketing them to the public.

Once the harmful health impacts of smoking became clear, antismoking advocates and public health organizations demanded that the FDA take steps to regulate tobacco products. The tobacco companies resisted such demands, however, by claiming that cigarettes did not fall under the agency's purview because they were neither consumed as food nor administered as therapeutic drugs. Upon assuming the position of FDA commissioner in 1990, Kessler launched an investigation of the tobacco industry. With the assistance of whistleblowers who provided confidential documents and research from inside the tobacco companies, the FDA uncovered evidence that cigarette manufacturers knew about the addictive capacity of nicotine, intentionally manipulated nicotine levels to increase the potential for addiction, and specifically marketed their products to underage youth.

In August 1996, the FDA officially claimed jurisdiction over tobacco products by defining nicotine as a drug and cigarettes as medical devices intended to deliver nicotine. Kessler declared that the agency had the authority to regulate the chemical composition of tobacco products as well as the labeling, marketing, and promotion practices employed by the tobacco industry. Led by Brown and Williamson Tobacco Corporation, a group of cigarette manufacturers challenged the FDA's regulatory authority in court. The tobacco companies claimed that their products did not qualify as "drugs" under the Food, Drug, and Cosmetic Act because cigarettes were not customarily marketed as providing therapeutic benefits to consumers. As the case of *Brown and Williamson v. FDA,* 529 U.S. 120 wound its way through the court system, the four largest American cigarette manufacturers agreed to settle civil lawsuits brought by state attorneys general. The 1998 settlement agreement required the tobacco companies to pay the states $246 billion in reimbursement for the public health costs associated with treating smoking-related illnesses.

Brown and Williamson v. FDA eventually reached the U.S. Supreme Court, which issued a 5–4 ruling in favor of the tobacco companies in March 2000. In the majority opinion, Justice Sandra Day O'Connor said that the FDA had overstepped its regulatory authority by asserting control over tobacco. "Congress, for better or for worse, has created a distinct regulatory scheme for tobacco products, squarely rejected proposals to give the FDA jurisdiction over tobacco, and repeatedly acted to preclude any agency from exercising significant policymaking authority in the area," she wrote. At the same time, O'Connor acknowledged the societal costs of tobacco use. "By no means do we question the seriousness of the problem that the FDA has sought to address," she noted. "The agency has amply demonstrated that tobacco use, particularly among children and adolescents, poses perhaps the single most significant threat to public health in the United States" (Biskupic 2000).

Congress Grants the FDA Authority to Regulate Tobacco

Kessler, who stepped down as FDA commissioner in 1997, expressed disappointment with the ruling and called on Congress to rectify the situation. Although proponents of tobacco control subsequently introduced several bills to grant the necessary regulatory authority to the FDA, the tobacco lobby and its allies in Congress managed to prevent their passage for nearly a decade. In the meantime, the U.S. Department of Justice (DOJ) launched a new lawsuit against the tobacco companies, accusing them of conspiring to deceive the public about the health risks of smoking and the addictive capacity of nicotine. In 2006, U.S. District Court Judge Gladys Kessler ruled in favor of the DOJ in *United States v. Philip Morris.* Her decision provided the government with legal remedies to prevent future violations by the tobacco companies, such as prohibiting certain marketing practices and compelling the release of "corrective statements" about the harmful health effects of smoking.

After President Barack Obama took office in 2009, antismoking advocates and public health officials viewed his administration's focus on health care as an opportunity to pass legislation giving the FDA jurisdiction over tobacco products. Representative Henry Waxman (D-CA), who led the questioning of U.S. tobacco executives during the famous 1994 congressional hearings on smoking and health, co-sponsored the Family Smoking Prevention and Tobacco Control Act. When Obama signed the bill into law on June 22, 2009, it overturned *Brown and Williamson v. FDA* and formally granted the FDA authority to regulate the content, manufacture, marketing, and sale of tobacco products in the United States.

The Tobacco Control Act includes many provisions aimed at reducing access to tobacco products by underage youth, including a ban on public vending-machine sales of cigarettes and a prohibition of tobacco company sponsorship of entertainment, sports, social, and cultural events. The legislation also increases the size of cigarette warning labels to cover 50 percent of the front and back of packaging. Although the FDA originally mandated graphic health warnings with pictorial depictions of the negative health consequences of smoking—such as blackened lungs, a mouth full of cancerous lesions, or an infant enveloped in a cloud of cigarette smoke—the tobacco industry successfully challenged this provision in court, arguing that the graphic warnings violated cigarette makers' First Amendment rights by forcing them to participate in antismoking advocacy.

The Tobacco Control Act created a new entity within the FDA, the Center for Tobacco Products, to regulate the content of tobacco products. The legislation requires manufacturers to disclose all product ingredients and allows the FDA to inspect production facilities and establish product standards—including reducing, but not eliminating, nicotine. It also bans the use of flavorings in cigarettes, with the exception of menthol. Finally, the act requires manufacturers to obtain FDA approval before introducing new tobacco products and to provide scientific evidence before making "modified risk" health claims (such as "light," "low-tar," or "mild") in tobacco advertising. The Tobacco Control Act also imposes some limitations on the agency's regulatory authority. The law prohibits the FDA from banning entire classes of tobacco products or requiring manufacturers to remove all nicotine. It also prohibits the agency from requiring prescriptions for tobacco purchases, raising the minimum age for tobacco purchases above 18 years, and banning tobacco sales from specific types of retail outlets.

Assessment of the Tobacco Control Act

The Tobacco Control Act received support from nearly 1,000 antismoking organizations and public health groups, including the American Cancer Society and the American Heart Association. Supporters praised the legislation for requiring tobacco companies to disclose all the harmful ingredients in their products and for enacting measures to prevent young people from smoking. Some antismoking advocates argued that the law did not go far enough, however, because it did not allow the FDA to ban cigarettes or eliminate nicotine. They asserted that reducing the level of nicotine in cigarettes would be ineffective because consumers would compensate by inhaling more deeply or smoking more cigarettes to satisfy their cravings.

Some critics opposed the Tobacco Control Act because lobbyists for tobacco industry leader Philip Morris played a role in crafting the legislation. Following the massive financial settlement to conclude the state litigation, Philip Morris and its parent company, Altria, shifted their strategy toward shaping government regulation to create a more stable and predictable business environment. Concern that the cigarette maker exerted influence over its provisions prompted some opponents of the law to derisively call it the "Marlboro Protection Act" or "Marlboro Monopoly Act." Critics saw evidence of the company's influence in the law's exception for menthol-flavored cigarettes as well as its regulatory barriers against the introduction of new products. "It is a dream come true for Philip Morris," said public health expert Michael Siegel. "First, they make it look like they are a reformed company which really cares about reducing the toll of cigarettes and protecting the public's health; and second, they protect their domination of the market and make it impossible for potentially competitive products to enter" (Smalera 2009).

Electronic cigarette manufacturers and vaping enthusiasts also expressed concerns about FDA regulation of the tobacco industry. They worried that e-cigarettes would be subject to the FDA's premarket approval process for new or reduced-harm tobacco products, which would create financial burdens for small manufacturers. They also questioned whether the ban on flavored tobacco would apply to e-liquid flavors. Although advocates of vaping viewed e-cigarettes as safer alternatives for nicotine delivery, they claimed that the law placed newer technological developments at a significant disadvantage compared to conventional cigarettes.

Further Reading

Biskupic, Joan. 2000. "FDA Can't Regulate Tobacco, Supreme Court Rules 5–4." *Washington Post,* March 20, 2000. https://www.washingtonpost.com /archive/politics/2000/03/22/fda-cant-regulate-tobacco-supreme-court -rules-5-to-4/3e3fd725-a469-4261-b660-a3415d2f99c1.

McDaniel, P. A., and R. E. Malone. 2005. "Understanding Philip Morris's Pursuit of U.S. Government Regulation of Tobacco." *Tobacco Control* 14 (3): 193– 200, May 27, 2005. https://tobaccocontrol.bmj.com/content/14/3/193.

Nelson, Steve. 2014. "House Leaders Rush to Defend E-Cigarettes from Possible FDA Bans." *U.S. News and World Report,* December 3, 2014. https://www .usnews.com/news/articles/2014/12/03/house-leaders-rush-to-defend -e-cigarettes-from-possible-fda-bans.

Smalera, Paul. 2009. "Cool, Refreshing Legislation for Philip Morris." *Slate,* June 8, 2009. http://blogs.reuters.com/great-debate/2009/06/12/cool-refres hing-legislation-for-philip-morris/.

U.S. Food and Drug Administration. 2018. "Family Smoking Prevention and Tobacco Control Act—An Overview." https://www.fda.gov/TobaccoProd ucts/GuidanceComplianceRegulatoryInformation/ucm246129.htm.

Wilson, Duff. 2009. "Philip Morris's Support Casts Shadow over a Bill to Limit Tobacco." *New York Times,* March 31, 2009. https://www.nytimes.com /2009/04/01/business/01tobacco.html.

Federal Courts Define E-Cigarettes as Tobacco Products (2010)

In response to the 2009 warning issued by the World Health Organization (WHO) and concerns expressed by other public health experts, the U.S. Food and Drug Administration (FDA) sought to restrict the sale of electronic cigarettes in the United States. Agency officials questioned the safety of the new devices, which had been introduced to American consumers without extensive testing, as well as elements of product design and marketing that seemed to target children. The FDA's efforts to regulate e-cigarettes received strong support from antismoking advocates. Although some manufacturers presented e-cigarettes as reduced-harm alternatives that could help people quit smoking, tobacco-control groups warned that vaping also had the potential to attract nonsmokers and cause them to become addicted to nicotine.

The FDA Defines E-Cigarettes as Drug-Delivery Devices

From the time e-cigarettes first appeared, public health officials debated about how to classify them for regulatory purposes. The FDA initially claimed jurisdiction by defining e-cigarettes as drug-delivery systems intended for the medical treatment of nicotine addiction. This definition equated vaping with nicotine replacement therapies (NRTs)—such as gum, patches, or inhalers—used as smoking-cessation tools, which fell under the FDA's broad authority to regulate therapeutic drugs and medical devices. In April 2009, the FDA used this rationale to prevent shipments of e-cigarettes and accessories manufactured by Smoking Everywhere from entering the United States. In addition, several states and municipalities took steps to ban the sale of e-cigarettes, enact age restrictions to prevent access by minors, or prohibit vaping in public places.

Smoking Everywhere immediately asked the U.S. District Court for the District of Columbia to grant a preliminary injunction blocking the FDA order from taking effect until its legality could be determined. Along with Sottera Inc., producer of the NJOY e-cigarette brand, Smoking Everywhere filed a lawsuit challenging the FDA's regulatory authority. The manufacturers argued that their products were not intended to provide medical treatment for nicotine addiction. Instead, they asserted that e-cigarettes were designed to deliver nicotine for users' recreational enjoyment. This definition placed e-cigarettes in the same category as traditional cigarettes and other tobacco products, which were not subject to FDA regulation at that time.

As *Smoking Everywhere v. FDA* proceeded through the legal system, it generated intense interest from antismoking advocates and vaping enthusiasts alike. Many public health groups filed amicus briefs in support of the FDA's position, including the American Academy of Pediatrics, American Cancer Society, American Heart Association, American Medical Association, and Campaign for Tobacco-Free Kids. Proponents of e-cigarettes, on the other hand, portrayed them as reduced-harm alternatives that had the potential to reduce smoking-related diseases and benefit public health. "Cigarette smoking remains the leading cause of preventable disease and death in the United States today," declared Elizabeth Whelan, a physician and president of the American Council on Science and Health. "Any alternative acceptable to addicted smokers should be taken seriously. Instead of condemning the e-cigarette, the FDA should be sponsoring studies to evaluate its safety and efficacy—leaving it on the market in the interim" (Whelan 2009). Several trade groups filed amicus briefs in support of Smoking Everywhere, including the Electronic Cigarette Association, Consumer Advocates for Smoke-Free Alternatives Association, and the National Vapers Club.

The Courts Change the Definition

While the case was ongoing, Congress passed the Family Smoking Prevention and Tobacco Control Act, which granted the FDA authority to regulate tobacco products. The law defined a tobacco product as "any product made or derived from tobacco that is intended for human consumption, including any component, part, or accessory of a tobacco product." On January 14, 2010, Judge Richard Leon of the U.S. District Court issued a ruling in favor of Smoking Everywhere and Sottera. Leon granted the companies an injunction, which allowed them to continue importing and selling e-cigarettes in the United States. He also interpreted the Tobacco Control Act to mean that e-cigarettes should be classified as modified-risk tobacco products rather than drug-delivery devices.

The FDA appealed the ruling, and the U.S. Court of Appeals for the D.C. Circuit heard oral arguments in the case in September 2010. Three months later, Judge Stephen Williams affirmed the lower court's judgment that the FDA had the authority to regulate e-cigarettes as tobacco products only if they were marketed as providing therapeutic benefits to users. In April 2011, the FDA declined to pursue the case further and agreed to abide by the ruling. Craig Weiss, president of Sottera, called the decision "enormously satisfying" for the entire vaping industry. "We very much look forward to working with the FDA on a going-forward basis to help shape and promulgate the regulations that are forthcoming," he added (Zid 2011).

The Tobacco Control Act authorized the FDA to issue regulations "deeming" specific tobacco products subject to restrictions that are intended to protect public health. Following the *Smoking Everywhere v. FDA* ruling, antismoking advocates and public health organizations began pressuring the FDA to deem e-cigarettes subject to the same regulations as other tobacco products. Although the law prohibited the FDA from banning entire classes of tobacco products or requiring manufacturers to remove all nicotine, it gave the agency broad authority to establish product standards and restrict advertising.

In the meantime, some early studies suggested e-cigarettes offered potential health benefits as smoking-cessation tools. Articles appearing in such reputable sources as the *American Journal of Preventive Medicine, Addiction,* and *BMC Public Health* reported that e-cigarettes were more effective than FDA-approved NRT products in helping research subjects cut down or quit smoking cigarettes. Proponents of vaping seized upon such reports to argue that public health officials should embrace e-cigarettes as reduced-harm alternatives to combustible cigarettes. Under the *Smoking Everywhere v. FDA* ruling, however, e-cigarette manufacturers could not market their products as smoking-cessation tools without risking strict government regulation as drug-delivery devices.

The definition of e-cigarettes as tobacco products became even more complicated as some manufacturers began using synthetic nicotine in vape juice. Although trace amounts of nicotine occur naturally in several varieties of plants—including tomatoes, peppers, and eggplant—the chemical is highly concentrated in the tobacco plant, so most nicotine is extracted from tobacco. The definition of e-cigarettes as tobacco products under the Tobacco Control Act was based on the fact that e-liquid is "derived from tobacco." Within a few years after the first e-cigarettes appeared in the United States, however, such companies as Next Generation Labs perfected the process of synthesizing nicotine without tobacco, raising further questions about FDA jurisdiction.

Further Reading

Family Smoking Prevention and Tobacco Control Act. 2009. Congress.gov. https://www.congress.gov/bill/111th-congress/house-bill/1256/text?overview=closed.

Whelan, Elizabeth. 2009. "FDA Smokescreen on E-Cigarettes." *Washington Times,* August 6, 2009. https://www.washingtontimes.com/news/2009/aug/06/fda-smoke-screen-on-e-cigarettes/.

Zhang, Sarah. 2016. "E-Cigs Are Going Tobacco-Free with Synthetic Nicotine." Wired, June 26, 2016. https://www.wired.com/2016/06/vaping-industry-wants-go-post-tobacco-synthetic-nicotine/.

Zid, Linda Abu-Shalback. 2011. "Up Next for Sottera." *CSP,* May 3, 2011. https://www.cspdailynews.com/tobacco/next-sottera.

The Debate over the Health Risks of Vaping (2014)

After federal courts ruled that the U.S. Food and Drug Administration (FDA) could regulate electronic cigarettes as tobacco products under the Family Smoking Prevention and Tobacco Control Act of 2009, vaping supporters and opponents waited to see what steps the agency would take next. Until the FDA finalized its "deeming" rules for e-cigarettes, though, the vaping industry went largely unregulated for several years. Most e-cigarette manufacturers carefully avoided making overt health claims to prevent their products from being reclassified as drug-delivery systems. In other ways, however, their marketing strategies pushed far beyond the limits that federal regulators had spent decades fighting to establish for conventional cigarettes. E-cigarette advertisements—often featuring celebrity endorsements—appeared on television, in print media, and on the Internet. Sellers of e-cigarettes also raised brand awareness by sponsoring scholarship competitions, concerts, film festivals, and sporting events.

Along with the introduction of sleek, high-tech product designs and appealing flavors, these advertising campaigns helped create a perception of e-cigarettes as cool, fun, exciting, and sexy. As a result, their popularity expanded rapidly. By 2015, less than a decade after e-cigarettes reached the U.S. market, an estimated 20 million American adults had tried vaping (Venton 2015). Many vapers were former smokers who used e-cigarettes to reduce their consumption of traditional cigarettes or to quit smoking altogether. They promoted vaping as a reduced-harm alternative to combustible cigarettes and provided anecdotal evidence of dramatic health improvements that they attributed to e-cigarettes. Vaping enthusiasts formed user groups, such as the American Vaping Association and NOT Blowing Smoke, that vocally defended e-cigarettes against criticism and actively opposed government regulation. "There is this hyper-aggressive social media response to anyone who doesn't think e-cigarettes are the greatest things ever," said tobacco-control advocate Stanton Glantz. "They're trying to shut down any criticism" (Venton 2015).

At the same time, the growing popularity of vaping raised concerns among public health organizations and antismoking advocates. Critics pointed out that e-cigarettes had been introduced to American consumers without formal research or testing to prove the products' safety and efficacy. Others worried that the slick advertising campaigns would encourage young people and nonsmokers to try vaping, exposing them to nicotine addiction and undermining antismoking efforts. Many public health groups issued policy statements warning about potential health hazards associated with vaping and calling on the FDA to regulate the manufacture and sale of e-cigarettes. "E-cig people would like you to believe that because the evidence that we have on them is limited, that we don't know anything. And that's just not true," Glantz stated. "We already know you're breathing in a lot of toxic chemicals, which is bad. You're breathing in a lot of toxic particles, which is bad. You're taking in nicotine, which is bad. A cigarette is by far and away the most dangerous consumer product ever invented. So to say it's not as bad as a cigarette is not saying very much" (Venton 2015).

Public Health Experts Oppose Vaping

In 2014, several prominent medical journals and public health organizations weighed in on the contentious debate over the safety of e-cigarettes.

While some critics acknowledged that using e-cigarettes was likely to be less harmful than smoking regular cigarettes, they also asserted that vaping was unlikely to be harmless and demanded that it be studied and regulated. The American Heart Association (AHA)—a longtime supporter of tobacco-control laws and smoking-cessation programs—issued a policy statement in the journal *Circulation* urging the FDA to subject e-cigarettes to the same regulations as combustible cigarettes. Although the AHA noted that vaping provided a potential opportunity for harm reduction if smokers substituted e-cigarettes for regular cigarettes, the statement warned that the public health impact would be limited if nonsmokers took up vaping. AHA researchers found that American consumers had access to 466 brands of e-cigarettes and 7,764 unique flavors by early 2014 (Bhatnagar 2014). They expressed concern that vaping could increase nicotine addiction, normalize smoking, and reverse the progress of tobacco-control campaigns. They called on the FDA to reduce the negative health impacts by establishing product standards, requiring warning labels, imposing taxes, and prohibiting the marketing and sale of e-cigarettes to minors.

The American Academy of Pediatrics (AAP)—a professional organization representing 67,000 physicians dedicated to optimizing the health of children and adolescents—also issued a statement urging the FDA to claim regulatory authority over e-cigarettes. Based on a 2014 study suggesting that more young people used e-cigarettes than any other tobacco product, the AAP recommended implementing age restrictions for purchases, imposing bans on flavors that appealed to youth, and expanding smoke-free laws to cover vapor products. The organization also encouraged the vaping industry to adopt child-resistant packaging to prevent accidental exposure of children to liquid nicotine, a toxicant that prompted more than 3,000 calls to U.S. poison control centers in 2014 (Walley and Jenssen 2015).

Despite testimonials by vaping supporters who credited e-cigarettes with helping them quit smoking, some public health experts argued that the technology's tendency to cause nicotine addiction among nonsmokers outweighed its potential benefits as a smoking-cessation tool. In a survey of middle- and high-school students, the U.S. Centers for Disease Control and Prevention found that 263,000 respondents who had never smoked a conventional cigarette used e-cigarettes in 2013. The young people who experimented with vaping were more than twice as likely as their non-smoking peers to say they intended to smoke conventional cigarettes (CDC Newsroom 2014). "What I find most concerning about the rise of vaping is that people who would've never smoked otherwise, especially youth, are taking up the habit," said Michael J. Blaha of the Johns

Hopkins School of Medicine. "It's one thing if you convert from cigarette smoking to vaping. It's quite another thing to start up nicotine use with vaping. And, it often leads to using traditional tobacco products down the road" (Blaha 2019).

The *New England Journal of Medicine* confirmed this analysis in a study that described e-cigarettes as "gateway drugs," suggesting that they not only created nicotine addiction but increased users' susceptibility to other addictive substances. Another study, published in the *International Journal of Hygiene and Environmental Health,* raised new concerns about the potential health effects of secondhand exposure to nicotine vapor. The researchers found that vaping negatively affected indoor air quality by releasing particulate matter, aluminum, and other compounds that have been linked to lung diseases. Although e-cigarette vapor appeared to be significantly less harmful than secondhand cigarette smoke, public health experts noted that the long-term health effects remained unknown. In addition, critics worried that social acceptance of vaping in places where smoking was not allowed would undermine the long, hard-fought anti-smoking campaign. Swayed by the reports of health risks, many cities and states began restricting the sale of e-cigarettes or banning their use in public places.

Vaping Advocates Fight Back

E-cigarette manufacturers, retailers, and trade groups responded by claiming that the health concerns were overblown. They questioned the methodology of the scientific studies that found harmful effects of vaping and sponsored research that yielded contradictory results. For instance, one study claimed that propylene glycol and glycerin—common food additives used in e-liquids—degraded into toxic chemicals such as formaldehyde when heated and vaporized. Vaping supporters argued that the results were flawed because the researchers used much higher temperatures than those produced by the heating coils in e-cigarettes. They compared the study to toasting a piece of bread until it turned black and then claiming that the toaster produced carcinogens (Tolentino 2018).

While admitting that further research was needed to prove the long-term safety of vaping, supporters emphasized the immediate public health gains that might be realized by switching cigarette smokers to e-cigarettes. "Thirteen hundred people die from smoking every day," said David Abrams, an expert in public health and tobacco policy at New York University. "Imagine three jumbo jets crashing every single day with no survivors. But because this happens slowly and quietly, thirty or forty years after people start smoking, we no longer notice and we no longer care" (Tolentino 2018). A Georgetown University study estimated that switching 10 percent of American smokers to e-cigarettes each year for a decade would save 6.6 million lives (Tolentino 2018).

Proponents argued that the harm-reduction capacity of vaping outweighed its potential to cause nicotine addiction. They claimed that the historic association of nicotine with combustible cigarettes—and the deceptive practices of the tobacco industry—generated unwarranted concerns about its health effects. "Cigarettes were a wolf in sheep's clothing," Abrams acknowledged. "Now, with vaping, we have a sheep in wolf's clothing, and we cannot get the wolf out of our minds" (Tolentino 2018). Some vaping supporters compared nicotine to caffeine—a popular plant-based chemical stimulant that the FDA considers safe. "Chemically, nicotine is very similar to caffeine, and coffee is one of the most widely traded products in the world," said James Monsees, co-inventor of the Juul e-cigarette. "While people of all ages around the world enjoy coffee, nicotine has been heavily stigmatized" (Lee 2018).

Vaping supporters asserted that public health officials should embrace e-cigarettes as a safer alternative to conventional cigarettes rather than placing restrictions on their sale and use. "I'm afraid that we will look back at this moment and see that we had this unbelievable discovery, this technology that had the potential to put the final nail in the coffin in cigarette smoking in this country," said tobacco-control expert Michael Siegel, "and because of this ideology that nicotine itself should be prohibited, that anything that looks like smoking is bad, we will squander this opportunity, and we'll have gone back to where we were" (Tolentino 2018).

Further Reading

Bhatnagar, Aruni, et al. 2014. "Electronic Cigarettes: A Policy Statement from the American Heart Association." *Circulation* 130: 1418–1436. https://www.ahajournals.org/doi/pdf/10.1161/CIR.0000000000000107.

Blaha, Michael J. 2019. "Five Truths You Need to Know about Vaping." Johns Hopkins Medicine. https://www.hopkinsmedicine.org/health/healthy_heart/know_your_risks/5-truths-you-need-to-know-about-vaping.

CDC Newsroom. 2014. "More Than a Quarter-Million Youth Who Had Never Smoked a Cigarette Used E-Cigarettes in 2013." Centers for Disease Control and Prevention, August 25, 2014. https://www.cdc.gov/media/releases/2014/p0825-e-cigarettes.html.

Lee, Seung. 2018. "Juul Labs Co-Founders Say They're Working toward a World without Smokers." *San Jose Mercury News,* September 12, 2018. https://

www.mercurynews.com/2018/09/12/juul-labs-co-founders-say-theyre
-working-toward-a-world-without-smokers/.

Tolentino, Jia. 2018. "The Promise of Vaping and the Rise of Juul." *New Yorker,*
May 14, 2018. https://www.newyorker.com/magazine/2018/05/14/the
-promise-of-vaping-and-the-rise-of-juul.

Venton, Danielle. 2015. "The War over Vaping's Health Risks Is Getting Dirty."
Wired, April 2, 2015. https://www.wired.com/2015/04/war-vapings
-health-risks-getting-dirty/.

Walley, Susan C., and Brian P. Jenssen. 2015. "Electronic Nicotine Delivery Systems." *Pediatrics* 136 (5): 1018. http://pediatrics.aappublications.org/content
/136/5/1018.

Juul Increases the Popularity of Vaping (2015)

After electronic cigarettes appeared in the United States in 2007, sales
of the devices grew slowly at first, driven largely by cigarette smokers who
viewed vaping as a reduced-harm alternative for nicotine delivery. The
market began expanding in the early 2010s as hobbyists introduced mod-
ifications to improve the devices' appearance and function and large
tobacco companies developed competing products, such as blu (Loril-
lard/Imperial Tobacco), Logic (Japan Tobacco), MarkTen (Altria), and
Vuse (R. J. Reynolds). With the ongoing product innovation, the U.S.
Centers for Disease Control and Prevention (CDC) reported that sales of
e-cigarettes at retail outlets grew by 132 percent from 2012 to 2016 (Shapiro 2018).

In June 2015, a San Francisco–based technology startup introduced a
revolutionary new e-cigarette design called the Juul. The creators of the
device, Adam Bowen and James Monsees, met as graduate students in product design at Stanford University. After completing their master's degrees,
they launched a series of companies called Ploom, Pax Labs, and Juul Labs
in their quest to develop a nicotine-delivery system so appealing that it
would replace combustible cigarettes. "Our company's mission is to eliminate cigarettes and help the more than one billion smokers worldwide switch
to a better alternative," said Juul Labs CEO Kevin Burns (Belluz 2018).

Juul differed from e-cigarettes already on the market in several ways. It
was more compact in size and had a sleek, high-tech design that was often
compared to a computer flash drive. The main part of the device contained a heating element and a rechargeable battery that could be plugged
into a USB port. The system worked by vaporizing e-liquid contained in
replaceable cartridges known as pods that users inserted into the end of
the device. Juul pods contained a much higher concentration of nicotine,

at 59 milligrams per milliliter of liquid, than most other e-cigarettes. In addition, Juul pods used a unique combination of nicotine salts (protonated nicotine) and benzoic acid, which reduced the harshness of the inhaled vapor and increased the rate of absorption into the user's lungs and brain. As a result, the Juul delivered a fast-acting, potent nicotine hit that closely resembled the experience of smoking a cigarette.

Juul Experiences Explosive Growth

Juul quickly built a devoted following among cigarette smokers who sought a less harmful alternative. Supporters pointed out that smoking-related diseases killed nearly half a million Americans each year, and they touted Juul as an effective smoking-cessation tool. Scott Gottlieb, who was appointed FDA commissioner in 2017 by President Donald Trump, initially expressed optimism that Juul and other e-cigarettes could benefit public health by helping people quit smoking. "Two-thirds of adult smokers have stated they want to quit," he said. "They know it's hard, and they've probably tried many times to quit. We must recognize the potential for innovation to lead to less harmful products" (Richtel and Kaplan 2018).

Between 2016 and 2017, sales of Juul e-cigarettes increased by 614 percent, from 2.2 million units to 16.2 million units. Juul's sales tripled in 2018, and by the end of the year the company controlled three-quarters of the U.S. e-cigarette market (Richtel and Kaplan 2018). It soon became clear, however, that the product's popularity among teenagers fueled Juul's remarkable growth. Besides helping existing cigarette smokers to quit, Juul appeared to be enticing young people to experiment with vaping and risk becoming addicted to nicotine. In fact, the brand became so established among teenagers that they began to use "Juuling" as a verb in reference to vaping. High-school administrators across the United States reported students Juuling in bathroom stalls, hallways, and classrooms.

Public health officials grew alarmed at the rapid increase in teen vaping. Among high-school seniors, cigarette-smoking rates declined steadily for two decades, from 36.5 percent in 1997 to 7.6 percent in 2018. Anti-smoking advocates viewed the drop as evidence that their long struggle to regulate the tobacco industry and educate young people about the health risks of smoking had paid off. Then, following the introduction of Juul, vaping rates among 12th graders more than doubled within a single year, from 11 percent in 2017 to 26.7 percent in 2018 (Belluz 2018). Tobacco-control groups expressed concern that the surge in youth vaping would cause a new generation to become addicted to nicotine. They worried about the potential health risks associated with e-cigarettes as well as the possibility that teenagers who experimented with vaping would be more likely to smoke cigarettes. "I don't want anyone to think I'm against the harm-reduction potential of these devices for adults," U.S. Surgeon General Jerome Adams said in calling for increased regulation of e-cigarettes. "But 3 percent of adults are using these devices—[and] 20 percent of high schoolers are using these devices" (Belluz 2018).

The FDA Launches an Investigation

Concerns about underage use of e-cigarettes prompted the FDA to investigate Juul's product design and marketing strategies in an effort to understand its appeal to teenagers. Critics claimed that Juul's initial advertising campaign, "Vaporized," seemed intentionally designed to target young people by presenting Juuling as fun, trendy, and sexy. "Juul ads are filled with attractive young models socializing and flirtatiously sharing the flash-drive shaped device, displaying behavior like dancing to club-like music and clothing styles more characteristic of teens than mature adults," according to *Forbes* writer Kathleen Chaykowski (2018a). These colorful ads appeared in teen-oriented magazines and on social media platforms with large teen user bases, such as Instagram. Some critics saw similarities to cigarette ads that had appeared before federal advertising bans took effect. Vince Wilmore, a spokesperson for the Campaign for Tobacco-Free Kids, asserted that Juul "used the same imagery and themes that tobacco companies have always used to appeal to kids, and they fueled it with social media" (Tobin 2018).

The FDA investigation found that young people liked Juul's attractive design and resemblance to a computer memory stick, which made it less conspicuous to parents or teachers. Teenagers were also attracted by the compact size of the Juul device, which made it easy to conceal in a pocket, purse, or backpack. The availability of Juul pods with sweet flavors—such as mango, fruit, crème, and mint—also held appeal for underage users. The combination of these factors convinced several state attorneys general to file lawsuits against Juul for allegedly designing and marketing tobacco products to minors. "From our perspective, this is not about getting adults to stop smoking," said Massachusetts Attorney General Maura Healey. "This is about getting kids to start vaping, and [to] make money and have them as customers for life" (Richtel and Kaplan 2018).

Some tobacco-control advocates accused Juul of intentionally raising nicotine levels to create dependency while misleading consumers about the risks of addiction. A 2017 survey conducted by the antismoking advocacy organization Truth Initiative revealed that 63 percent of young people between the ages of 15 and 24 who used a Juul did not understand that the device delivered nicotine (Truth Initiative 2018). "In some cases, our kids are trying these products and liking them without even knowing they contain nicotine," Gottlieb stated. "And that's a problem, because as we know the nicotine in these products can rewire an adolescent's brain, leading to years of addiction" (Gottlieb 2018).

Juul executives responded to the criticism by insisting that they did not want their products to be used by minors. "We are committed to deterring young people, as well as adults who do not currently smoke, from using our products," said Burns. "We cannot be more emphatic on this point: No young person or non-nicotine user should ever try Juul" (Belluz 2018). The company announced plans to cooperate with the FDA and to spend $30 million on measures to reduce youth access to its products. Juul removed popular sweet flavors from retail stores, strengthened age-verification methods for online sales, and changed its advertising to feature testimonials by adults who quit smoking cigarettes with the help of Juul. The company's founders also expressed support for a national plan to increase the minimum age for purchasing vaping products from 18 to 21. Vaping enthusiasts criticized some of these measures, arguing that they would restrict the reduced-harm alternatives available to adult smokers while doing little to deter young people from Juuling.

By responding aggressively to concerns about underage vaping, Juul executives hoped to avoid stricter FDA regulation of e-cigarettes, along the lines of the regulations imposed on cigarette manufacturers under the Family Smoking Prevention and Tobacco Control Act of 2009. At the same time, though, the success of Juul attracted attention from the big tobacco companies, which were forced to recognize the threat to cigarette sales as more smokers switched to vaping. Some big tobacco companies responded by expanding their e-cigarette product lines and investing in profitable e-cigarette manufacturers.

In 2018, for instance, Altria—producer of the industry-leading Marlboro cigarette brand—spent $12.8 billion to purchase a 35 percent stake in Juul Labs. Critics described the decision to join forces with Altria as a "deal with the devil" that destroyed Juul's credibility as a company committed to harm reduction and public health. "Juul partnering with Altria," declared Truth Initiative CEO Robin Koval, "proves they are not in the business of saving lives and never have been" (Tiku 2018). Juul executives defended the deal and insisted that it would not detract from the company's mission. "We understand the controversy and skepticism that comes with an affiliation and partnership with the largest tobacco company in the U.S.," said Burns. "We were skeptical as well. But over the course of the last several months we were convinced by actions, not words, that in fact this partnership could help accelerate our success switching adult smokers" (Chaykowski 2018b).

Further Reading

Belluz, Julia. 2018. "Juul, the Vape Device Teens Are Getting Hooked On, Explained." Vox, December 20, 2018. https://www.vox.com/science-and -health/2018/5/1/17286638/juul-vaping-e-cigarette.

Chaykowski, Kathleen. 2018a. "The Disturbing Focus of Juul's Early Marketing Campaigns." *Forbes,* December 18, 2018. https://www.forbes.com/sites /kathleenchaykowski/2018/11/16/the-disturbing-focus-of-juuls-early -marketing-campaigns/#4f7cc32414f9.

Chaykowski, Kathleen. 2018b. "New Altria Deal Makes Juul Cofounders Billion- aires." *Forbes,* December 20, 2018. https://www.forbes.com/sites/kathle enchaykowski/2018/12/20/new-altria-deal-makes-juul-cofounders -billionaires/#12479a6e5a67.

Gottlieb, Scott. 2018. "Statement from FDA Commissioner Scott Gottlieb, M.D., on New Enforcement Actions and a Youth Tobacco Prevention Plan to Stop Youth Use of, and Access to, JUUL and Other E-cigarettes." U.S. Food and Drug Administration, April 24, 2018. https://www.fda.gov /NewsEvents/Newsroom/PressAnnouncements/ucm605432.htm.

Richtel, Matt, and Sheila Kaplan. 2018. "Did Juul Lure Teenagers and Get 'Cus- tomers for Life'?" *New York Times,* August 27, 2018. https://www.nytimes .com/2018/08/27/science/juul-vaping-teen-marketing.html.

Shapiro, Nina. 2018. "Electronic Cigarette Sales Soar as a Door Opens for Teen Smokers." *Forbes,* October 26, 2018. https://www.forbes.com/sites/nina shapiro/2018/10/16/electronic-cigarette-sales-soar-as-a-door-opens -for-teen-smokers/#3ff135576b91.

Tiku, Nitasha. 2018. "Juul Sheds Its Anti-Smoking Cred and Embraces Big Tobacco." *Wired,* December 20, 2018. https://www.wired.com/story/juul -sheds-anti-smoking-cred-embraces-big-tobacco/.

Tobin, Ben. 2018. "FDA Targets E-Cigarettes Like Juul as Teachers Fear 'Epi- demic' Use by Students." *USA Today,* August 16, 2018. https://www.usa today.com/story/money/2018/08/16/juul-labs-back-school-teachers -e-cigarettes/917531002/.

Tolentino, Jia. 2018. "The Promise of Vaping and the Rise of Juul." *New Yorker,* May 14, 2018. https://www.newyorker.com/magazine/2018/05/14/the -promise-of-vaping-and-the-rise-of-juul.

Truth Initiative. 2018. "Behind the Explosive Growth of Juul." December 2018. https://truthinitiative.org/news/behind-explosive-growth-juul.

Yakowicz, Will. 2018. "Inside Juul: The Most Promising, and Controversial, Vape Company in America." *Inc.,* September 24, 2018. https://www.inc .com/will-yakowicz/2018-private-titans-juul-labs-vaporizer-nicotine -electronic-cigarettes.html.

The Food and Drug Administration Issues Deeming Regulations (2016)

The Family Smoking Prevention and Tobacco Control Act of 2009 gave the U.S. Food and Drug Administration (FDA) authority to regulate tobacco products. Although the law did not initially apply to electronic cigarettes, which had only recently been introduced in the United States, it included a provision allowing the FDA to deem other products containing nicotine to be tobacco products—and thus subject to restrictions intended to promote public health—in the future.

With the likelihood of FDA regulation looming, supporters and opponents of vaping engaged in vigorous debates in courtrooms, in the scientific research community, in the media, and in living rooms and classrooms. Vaping advocates emphasized the potential benefits of e-cigarettes as reduced-harm alternatives and smoking-cessation aids for adult smokers of combustible cigarettes. They demanded that the FDA preserve access to what they viewed as lifesaving products. Vaping opponents, on the other hand, expressed concerns about e-cigarettes' unproven safety record and potential to introduce young people to nicotine. They demanded that the FDA enact strict regulations on e-cigarettes to protect consumers from health risks. Meanwhile, in the absence of federal regulation, sales of vaping products grew rapidly, from $20 million in 2008 to $1.7 billion in 2014 (Hemmerich, Klein, and Berman 2017).

Proposed Rules Generate Debate

On April 24, 2014, the FDA released a Notice of Proposed Rulemaking that outlined deeming regulations for e-cigarettes. Some of the proposed regulations would require manufacturers to register products and provide lists of ingredients, establish a federal minimum age of 18 for the purchase of vaping products, prohibit the distribution of free samples, and place nicotine warning labels on packaging. The most controversial provision would require e-cigarette manufacturers to submit premarket tobacco applications for all vaping products, including components and parts. To receive FDA approval and remain on the market, e-cigarette manufacturers would have to conduct extensive tests to prove that their products were safe for consumers and beneficial to public health.

The proposed rules offered an exemption from the premarket approval requirement for tobacco products that had existed in substantially equivalent form prior to February 2007, the predicate date of the Tobacco Control Act. Although no vaping products qualified for the exemption, it applied to most cigarettes and other traditional tobacco products. "The Tobacco Control Act 'grandfathered' all cigarettes already available for sale, but created difficult barriers to any new products that might attempt to enter the market," according to an analyst for the website Vaping360. "The act effectively protected existing cigarette brands from future competition—not just from other cigarettes, but also from low-risk nicotine products that might threaten the tobacco companies down the road" (McDonald 2017).

After issuing the notice, the FDA opened a 90-day period for public comments to help shape the final rule. The agency received more than 135,000 comments on the proposal, many of which came from former cigarette smokers who credited e-cigarettes with improving their health. Many vaping supporters pointed out the inconsistency of allowing deadly cigarettes to remain on the market while erecting regulatory barriers against reduced-harm alternatives. "There is no evidence that public health would benefit if FDA imposes the Deeming Regulation," wrote tobacco harm reduction activist Bill Godshall (2015). "We should be reminded that public health measures remain well-grounded in the biomedical and behavioral sciences, with cigarette smoking remaining public enemy number one, the major cause of preventable disease, disability, and death in America. . . . Rather than pursue reflex-action to demonize, ban, regulate and/or tax, vaping should be recognized as a disease prevention public health intervention" (Sklaroff, Godshall, and Gambescia 2017).

Many vaping supporters focused their ire on the premarket approval process, arguing that it was so complex, time-consuming, and expensive that it would effectively put the vaping industry out of business. They claimed that the FDA rules put the interests of large tobacco companies and pharmaceutical firms above those of independent e-cigarette manufacturers, local vape shops, and consumers. Pro-vaping groups—such as the Consumer Advocates for Smoke-Free Alternatives Association (CASAA), the Smoke-Free Alternatives Trade Association (SFATA), the American Vaping Association, and NOT Blowing Smoke—worked to raise public awareness of the threat the proposed regulations posed to the vaping industry. Documentary filmmaker Aaron Biebert explored the controversy in his movie *A Billion Lives* (2016), which argued that the tobacco industry, pharmaceutical companies, government agencies, and anti-cancer charities were engaged in a corrupt scheme to suppress vaping as a potentially lifesaving alternative to cigarette smoking.

While the FDA processed the input and worked to finalize its deeming regulations, the popularity of vaping skyrocketed following the 2015 introduction of the Juul e-cigarette. With its sleek design, sweet flavors, high nicotine content, and savvy social media presence, Juul quickly claimed 75 percent of the U.S. market. Critics charged that Juul's sales were driven by its strong appeal to teenagers, and a flurry of articles reported an apparent surge in student vaping in schools across the country.

Such reports raised alarms among public health officials, who drew parallels between some of the tactics used by the unregulated vaping industry and those that had characterized the tobacco industry prior to the federal government crackdown. They claimed that advertising campaigns for Juul and other e-cigarettes intentionally targeted young people, for instance, to create a lasting market for vaping products. They also asserted that e-cigarette makers manipulated nicotine levels and delivery systems to maximize their addictive capacity, thus ensuring repeat customers. Finally, critics argued that the vaping industry promoted confusion and skepticism about scientific evidence and attempted to discredit independent studies associating e-cigarettes with harmful health effects. Vaping supporters claimed that they were only pointing out flaws in the underlying research. "Many of the people who are being paid to conduct the science have been knowingly and intentionally manipulating their results, omitting results, selectively cherry picking and basically misrepresenting their own findings because they're getting federal funding," Godshall stated (Gross 2017).

Questions about the vaping industry's business practices grew louder as the big tobacco companies increased their involvement by purchasing patents and investing in e-cigarette manufacturers. Some critics contended that the tobacco firms would take advantage of the lack of federal regulation over vaping products to advance their own interests, whether by using e-cigarette marketing channels to promote cigarette smoking, adjusting the nicotine delivery of e-cigarettes to reduce their effectiveness as smoking-cessation aids, or co-opting vaping's reputation for harm reduction to appear more socially responsible and gain influence with policymakers. As the big tobacco companies began to dominate e-cigarette production, doubts arose about vaping supporters' portrayal of the industry as underdog entrepreneurs and small businesses trying to end cigarette smoking and save lives.

FDA Asserts Regulatory Control over E-Cigarettes

The FDA released the final version of its deeming regulations on May 5, 2016. Effective August 8, 2016, the FDA claimed authority over all "components and parts" of vaping products, including "e-liquids; atomizers; batteries (with or without variable voltage); cartomizers (atomizer plus replaceable fluid-filled cartridge); digital display/lights to adjust settings; clearomizers, tank systems, flavors, vials that contain e-liquids, and programmable software" (FDA 2016). Any new devices, models, formulations, or flavors introduced after the effective date required submission and approval of a premarket tobacco application proving that they were "appropriate for the protection of public health." For existing vaping products already on the market, the deadline for completing the premarket approval process was August 8, 2018. Although the FDA issued a Guidance for Industry to assist e-cigarette manufacturers in preparing premarket applications, it did not provide specific technical or safety standards for them to meet to ensure approval.

In introducing the deeming rule, FDA Commissioner Robert M. Califf described it as a consumer-protection milestone. "At the FDA we must do our job under the Tobacco Control Act to reduce the harms caused by tobacco," he stated. "That includes ensuring consumers have the information they need to make informed decisions about tobacco use and making sure that new tobacco products for purchase come under comprehensive review" (Boyles 2016). A group of 17 Democratic senators sent a letter to Califf applauding the new regulations. "The deeming rule is a much-needed step to give the FDA crucial tools to prevent manufacturers and retailers of currently unregulated tobacco products from targeting our children and teens," they wrote, "and we urge your agencies to remain diligent in working quickly to further limit the effect and reach of these products on our nation's youth" (U.S. Senate Committee 2016).

To vaping supporters, however, the rules amounted to an attack on the booming e-cigarette industry and a blow to the cause of tobacco harm reduction and smoking-related disease prevention. CASAA issued a statement condemning the deeming rule, which it claimed would cripple the vaping industry and harm public health. "Rather than work toward supporting innovation of less harmful products, FDA's actions demonstrate a clear preference for the status quo, which keeps dangerous products in place while stifling their low-risk competitors," the statement said. "In no uncertain terms, the FDA regulations are an unmitigated disaster which will only increase suffering by prolonging the war on smoking" (Clark 2016). Several Republican members of Congress responded to these concerns by introducing legislation to adjust the predicate date in the Tobacco Control Act so that existing vaping products would be exempt from premarket approval requirements.

Vaping supporters and e-cigarette manufacturers also challenged the deeming regulations in court. The Right to Be Smoke-Free Coalition (R2BSF) trade group joined Nicopure Labs, maker of Halo brand e-liquids, in claiming that the FDA exceeded its jurisdiction and violated the vaping industry's First Amendment rights by preventing companies from marketing their products as reduced-harm alternatives to cigarettes. Critics noted that the law firm representing the vaping industry was the same one that tobacco giant Philip Morris had used to challenge and delay the implementation of laws protecting people from the dangers of secondhand smoke. In July 2017, U.S. District Court Judge Amy Berman Jackson ruled in favor of the FDA. "This provision does not ban truthful statements about health benefits or reduced risks," she said of the deeming rules, "it simply requires that they be substantiated" (Gross 2017).

A week later, however, newly installed FDA Commissioner Scott Gottlieb offered the vaping industry a reprieve from the deeming regulations. Gottlieb was appointed to the position by Republican President Donald Trump, and his background included positions with the conservative American Enterprise Institute—which expressed support for vaping as a reduced-harm alternative to combustible tobacco products—and on the board of directors of Kure, a vape shop franchise. On July 27, 2017, Gottlieb announced plans to postpone the premarket tobacco application deadline for existing e-cigarette products for four years, to August 8, 2022. He also promised to create clear standards and guidance for the approval process and to allow vaping products to remain on the market until the FDA completed its reviews.

Gottlieb described the changes as part of a comprehensive new FDA strategy for the regulation of nicotine, which included reducing the level of nicotine allowed in combustible cigarettes and providing smokers with reduced-harm alternatives. "We need to take a fresh look at nicotine itself, and how the addiction that it causes relates to the potential harm of its delivery mechanism," he stated. "We must acknowledge that there's a continuum of risk for nicotine delivery. That continuum ranges from combustible cigarettes at one end, to medicinal nicotine products at the other. . . . And we must recognize the potential for innovation to lead to less harmful products, which, under FDA's oversight, could be part of a solution. While there's still much research to be done on these products and the risks that they may pose, they may also present benefits that we must consider. . . . It's incumbent upon us as regulators to explore both the potential public health benefits and the risks of this new technology with an open mind" (Gottlieb 2017).

Pro-vaping groups applauded the change, claiming that it saved the e-cigarette industry as well as smokers' lives. They viewed it as the first of many needed reforms, however, and vowed to continue working to preserve consumer access to a variety of different devices and flavors. While antismoking advocates praised Gottlieb's proposal to reduce the level of nicotine in combustible tobacco products, they expressed concern that the policy left e-cigarettes unregulated for four more years. "I think FDA is being overly optimistic about the public health benefits of pushing people to switch," said tobacco-control expert Stanton Glantz. "If people switch to [e-cigarettes] and think they're safe, that's a real problem" (Becker 2017).

Further Reading

Becker, Rachel. 2017. "FDA's Plans for Low-Nicotine Cigarettes Could Drive More People to Vape." The Verge, July 28, 2017. https://www.theverge .com/2017/7/28/16060670/fda-low-nicotine-cigarettes-vape-e-cigs -regulation.

Boyles, Salynn. 2016. "FDA Regulates E-Cigarettes, Hookahs." MedPage Today, May 5, 2016. https://www.medpagetoday.com/pulmonology/smoking /57728.

Clark, Alex. 2016. "New FDA E-Cigarette Regulations Condemned by CASAA." Consumer Advocates for Smoke-free Alternatives Association, May 6, 2016. http://www.casaa.org/news/new-fda-e-cigarette-regulations-conde mned-by-casaa/.

FDA. 2016. "Rule Deeming Tobacco Products to Be Subject to the Federal Food, Drug, and Cosmetic Act, as Amended by the Family Smoking Prevention and Tobacco Control Act." *Federal Register*, May 10, 2016. https://www .federalregister.gov/documents/2016/05/10/2016-10685/deeming -tobacco-products-to-be-subject-to-the-federal-food-drug-and-cosmetic -act-as-amended-by-the.

Godshall, William T. 2015. "Comments to the FDA Center for Tobacco Products." Consumer Advocates for Smoke-free Alternatives Association, December 2015. http://www.casaa.org/wp-content/uploads/GodshallFD Acomment-December-2015.pdf.

Gottlieb, Scott. 2017. "Protecting American Families: Comprehensive Approach to Nicotine and Tobacco." U.S. Food and Drug Administration, July 28, 2017. https://www.fda.gov/NewsEvents/Speeches/ucm569024.htm.

Gross, Liza. 2017. "Smoke Screen: Big Vape Is Copying Big Tobacco's Playbook." The Verge, November 16, 2017. https://www.theverge.com/2017/11/16/166 58358/vape-lobby-vaping-health-risks-nicotine-big-tobacco-marketing.

Hemmerich, Natalie, Elizabeth G. Klein, and Micah Berman. 2017. "Evidentiary Support in Public Comments to the FDA's Center for Tobacco Products." *Journal of Health Politics, Policy, and Law* 42 (4): 645–666, August 1, 2017.

McDonald, Jim. 2019. "The Deeming Rule: A Brief History and Timeline of the FDA's Vaping Regulations." Vaping360, February 11, 2019. https://vaping 360.com/rules-laws/fda-deeming-regulations-timeline/.

Sklaroff, Robert, Bill Godshall, and Stephen F. Gambescia. 2017. "Vaping Isn't Smoking, It's a Disease-Prevention Method." *The Hill*, March 17, 2017. https://thehill.com/blogs/pundits-blog/healthcare/324534-vaping -should-be-recognized-as-a-disease-prevention-public.

U.S. Senate Committee on Health, Education, Labor, and Pensions. 2016. "Senate Dems: FDA Rule Is Critical Step to Protecting Children and Teens from Tobacco Products." Senate.gov, May 11, 2016. https://www.help.senate .gov/ranking/newsroom/press/senate-dems-fda-rule-is-critical-step-to -protecting-children-and-teens-from-tobacco-products-.

Youth Vaping Becomes an "Epidemic" (2018)

Electronic cigarette manufacturers and vaping enthusiasts expressed relief in 2017, when FDA Commissioner Scott Gottlieb announced plans to delay enforcement of the premarket tobacco application requirements for vaping products until 2022. His decision, which recognized vaping's harm-reduction potential for adult smokers of combustible cigarettes, allowed popular e-cigarette devices and flavors to remain on the market. Public health groups, on the other hand, expressed outrage about the postponement of federal regulation of the vaping industry. Led by the American Academy of Pediatrics, several health organizations filed a lawsuit against the FDA to demand immediate action on vaping. "It is illegal, unreasonable, and devastating for the public health for the FDA to postpone its oversight obligations any further," the American Medical Association stated in an amicus brief (Henry 2018).

In 2018, the regulatory landscape for vaping products shifted once again in response to evidence of the surging popularity of innovative e-cigarette brands such as Juul among teenagers. The National Youth Tobacco Survey found that 3.6 million American middle-school and high-school students reported using e-cigarettes during the past 30 days in 2018. Vaping rates reached 20.8 percent among high-school students, an increase of 78 percent from the previous year, and 11.7 percent among middle-school students, an increase of 48 percent from 2017 (Cullen et al. 2018). Antismoking advocates viewed these statistics with alarm. They argued that the strong appeal of vaping products to young people threatened to reverse decades of gains in tobacco control. "If you were to design your ideal nicotine-delivery device to addict large numbers of United States kids, you'd invent Juul," said Jonathan Winickoff, a pediatrician specializing in youth tobacco use. "It's absolutely unconscionable. The earlier these companies introduce the product to the developing brain, the better the chance they have a lifelong user" (Tolentino 2018).

The growing concerns about teen vaping led the FDA to implement a Youth Tobacco Prevention Program to restrict access, limit appeal, and reduce exposure to nicotine-containing products by minors. As part of the program, the agency launched a campaign called "The Real Cost" to educate young people about the risks of vaping and nicotine addiction. It featured a series of online video and radio messages on YouTube, Spotify, and other platforms popular with teenagers. The FDA also conducted investigations to determine how underage people were obtaining tobacco products. The results led to an "enforcement blitz" in which the agency issued warning citations or imposed fines on retailers that made illegal sales of vaping products to minors. The FDA also worked with the online retailer eBay to foreclose online sales of e-cigarettes to minors by third-party sellers. Finally, the agency examined the marketing practices of Juul and other e-cigarette manufacturers to determine whether they intentionally tried to appeal to youth. This investigation led the Federal Trade Commission to order several companies to cease using misleading, kid-friendly packaging that made vaping products look like candy, cookies, or juice.

Despite these measures, evidence continued to mount of a nationwide surge in youth vaping. Teachers and school administrators reported students vaping in hallways and bathrooms, and images and videos abounded on social media showing teenagers vaping outside of school. "Young people have taken a technology that was supposed to help grownups stop smoking and invented a new kind of bad habit, one that they have molded in their own image," Jia Tolentino wrote in the *New Yorker*. "The potential public-health benefit of the e-cigarette is being eclipsed by the unsettling prospect of a generation of children who may really love to vape" (Tolentino 2018). Public health experts asserted that early exposure to nicotine increased the risk of addiction and lifelong health problems, including anxiety, depression, and memory issues. "The adolescent brain is uniquely sensitive to nicotine and becomes addicted more rapidly and at lower concentrations," Winickoff explained. "The younger a teen starts smoking or vaping, the harder it will be to quit" (Becker 2018).

FDA Commissioner Declares an Epidemic

In September 2018, Gottlieb declared youth vaping an "epidemic" and threatened to take drastic action to prevent e-cigarette use by minors— even if that meant restricting adults' access to the full range of vaping devices and flavors. "I use the word epidemic with great care. E-cigs have become an almost ubiquitous—and dangerous—trend among teens. The disturbing and accelerating trajectory of use we're seeing in youth, and the resulting path to addiction, must end," the commissioner stated. "The FDA won't tolerate a whole generation of young people becoming addicted to nicotine as a tradeoff for enabling adults to have unfettered access to these same products. . . . It's now clear to me, that in closing the on-ramp to kids, we're going to have to narrow the off-ramp for adults who want to migrate off combustible tobacco and onto e-cigs" (Gottlieb 2018b).

Gottlieb warned the manufacturers of five e-cigarette brands that together controlled 97 percent of the U.S. market—Juul, Vuse, MarkTen, blu, and Logic—that he was reconsidering the FDA's approach to tobacco regulation in light of the youth vaping epidemic. He gave the companies 60 days to develop comprehensive plans to prevent minors from obtaining their products. If they failed to do so, Gottlieb threatened to halt sales of flavored e-liquids, which he said attracted underage users. He also suggested that the FDA might rescind its decision to extend the deadline for premarket tobacco applications until 2022 and begin enforcing the provision immediately, which would effectively take most vaping products off the market. "I've been warning the e-cigarette industry for more than a year that they needed to do much more to stem the youth trends," Gottlieb stated. "They say they've changed from the days of Joe Camel. But look at what's happening right now, on our watch and on their watch. They must demonstrate that they're truly committed to keeping these new products out of the hands of kids and they must find a way to reverse this trend. . . . We're at a crossroads today. It's one where the opportunities from new innovations will be responsibly seized on right now, or perhaps lost forever" (Gottlieb 2018b).

Public health and tobacco-control organizations praised Gottlieb's announcement. Matthew Myers, president of the Campaign for Tobacco-Free Kids, described it as "potentially the most important step FDA has taken to curtail youth use of e-cigarettes" (McGinley 2018). Robin Koval, chief executive of antismoking Truth Initiative, urged Gottlieb to follow through on his threat to make vaping products subject to immediate premarket approval. "Congress gave FDA all the authority and FDA has all the tools they need to regulate this market and they need to do this quickly," she stated. Koval questioned Gottlieb's decision to allow e-cigarette manufacturers to present plans for reducing youth vaping. Given the tobacco industry's long history of resisting federal regulation, she compared it to "asking the proverbial fox to guard the henhouse" (O'Donnell 2018).

Vaping supporters took issue with many aspects of the FDA commissioner's statement. Critics objected to Gottlieb's characterization of youth vaping as an "epidemic," calling it a charged term that was intended to provoke moral outrage over normal teen experimentation. They also questioned the FDA's interpretation of the data on youth vaping, arguing that high rates of e-cigarette use in the past 30 days did not necessarily mean that those teenagers were regular, daily vapers or addicted to nicotine. Critics further contended that concerns about youth vaping were overblown in comparison to other risky behavior by adolescents, noting that nearly 30 percent of high-school students reported using alcohol during the past 30 days in 2017, while 20 percent used marijuana, and 25 percent texted while driving (Kann, McManus, and Harris 2018).

Pro-vaping groups also pointed out that while the prevalence of youth vaping increased, the prevalence of youth cigarette smoking decreased, indicating that some teenagers were using e-cigarettes as a reduced-harm alternative or smoking-cessation tool. Finally, vaping supporters argued that restricting access to e-cigarettes and flavored e-liquids would harm public health by forcing adult vapers to use combustible cigarettes. "The FDA needs to be very cautious about the adverse effects that flavoring bans or excess regulation could have on this trend—smokers using vapor as a way to stop consuming cigarettes and move towards a healthier lifestyle," said Liz Mair, spokesperson for Vapers United (O'Donnell 2018).

In November 2018, leading e-cigarette producers Juul, Altria (Mark-Ten), Imperial Brands (blu), Japan Tobacco International (Logic), and British American Tobacco (Vuse) submitted proposals to the FDA for preventing youth vaping. Citing survey data showing that more than two-thirds of current high-school e-cigarette users preferred flavored vaping products, Gottlieb announced plans to prohibit the sale of flavored e-liquids at 90,000 retail outlets across the country, including grocery stores, drugstores, convenience stores, and gas stations. He said flavored pods would be available only at the 10,000 tobacco and vape shops nationwide that restricted access to customers over the age of 18. Under the plan, manufacturers that wanted to sell flavored products more broadly had to complete the premarket review process. "As a society, we've made great strides in stigmatizing cigarette use among kids. The kids using e-cigarettes are children who rejected conventional cigarettes, but don't see the same stigma associated with the use of e-cigarettes," Gottlieb stated. "I will not allow a generation of children to become addicted to nicotine through e-cigarettes. We must stop the trends of youth e-cigarette use from continuing to build and will take whatever action is necessary to ensure these kids don't become future smokers" (Gottlieb 2019).

Further Reading

Becker, Rachel. 2018. "Juul Is Being Investigated by Massachusetts for Hooking Kids on Vaping." The Verge, July 24, 2018. https://www.theverge.com/2018/7/24/17608136/juul-investigation-electronic-cigarettes-massachusetts-attorney-general-subpoena.

Cullen, Karen A., Bridget K. Ambrose, Andrea S. Gentzke, Benjamin J. Apelberg, Ahmed Jamal, and Brian A. King. 2018. "Notes from the Field: Use of Electronic Cigarettes and Any Tobacco Product among Middle and High School Students—United States, 2011–2018." *Morbidity and Mortality Weekly Report* 67 (45): 1276–1277, November 16, 2018. http://dx.doi.org/10.15585/mmwr.mm6745a5.

Gottlieb, Scott. 2018a. "Statement on New Enforcement Actions and a Youth Tobacco Prevention Plan to Stop Youth Use of, and Access to, JUUL and Other E-cigarettes." U.S. Food and Drug Administration, April 24, 2018. https://www.fda.gov/newsevents/newsroom/pressannouncements/ucm605432.htm.

Gottlieb, Scott. 2018b. "Statement on New Steps to Address Epidemic of Youth E-Cigarette Use." U.S. Food and Drug Administration, September 12, 2018. https://www.fda.gov/NewsEvents/Newsroom/PressAnnouncements/ucm620185.htm.

Gottlieb, Scott. 2019. "Statement on New Data Demonstrating Rising Youth Use of Tobacco Products and the Agency's Ongoing Actions to Confront the Epidemic of Youth E-Cigarette Use." U.S. Food and Drug Administration, February 11, 2019. https://www.fda.gov/NewsEvents/Newsroom/PressAnnouncements/ucm631112.htm.

Henry, Tanya A. 2018. "FDA Pulled into Federal Court on Delay in Regulating E-Cigarettes." American Medical Association, October 5, 2018. https://www.ama-assn.org/delivering-care/public-health/fda-pulled-federal-court-delay-regulating-e-cigarettes.

Kann, Laura, Tim McManus, and William A. Harris, et al. 2018. "Youth Risk Behavior Surveillance—United States, 2017. *Morbidity and Mortality Weekly Report* 67 (8): 1–114, June 15, 2018. https://www.cdc.gov/mmwr/volumes/67/ss/ss6708a1.htm.

McGinley, Laurie. 2018. "FDA Chief Calls Youth E-Cigarettes an 'Epidemic.'" *Washington Post,* September 12, 2018. https://www.washingtonpost.com/national/health-science/fda-chief-calls-youth-use-of-juul-other-e-cigarettes-an-epidemic/2018/09/12/.

O'Donnell, Jayne. 2018. "FDA Declares Youth Vaping an Epidemic, Announces Investigation, New Enforcement." *USA Today,* September 12, 2018. https://www.usatoday.com/story/news/politics/2018/09/12/fda-scott-gottlieb-youth-vaping-e-cigarettes-epidemic-enforcement/1266923002/.

Tolentino, Jia. 2018. "The Promise of Vaping and the Rise of Juul." *New Yorker,* May 14, 2018. https://www.newyorker.com/magazine/2018/05/14/the-promise-of-vaping-and-the-rise-of-juul.

CHAPTER THREE

Impacts of the Vaping Controversy

This chapter examines the impact of electronic cigarettes and vaping on specific areas of American life and culture. It outlines the struggle to control vaping in schools, explores the intersection of vaping and youth culture, and analyzes global approaches to tobacco control and e-cigarette regulation. It also examines the impact of vaping on the tobacco industry and on U.S. politics and public health.

Vaping in Schools

The prevalence of youth vaping in the United States first became clear in reports from teachers and administrators in the nation's schools. Years of antismoking campaigns helped reduce the rate of cigarette smoking among high-school students from 15.8 percent in 2011 to 8.1 percent in 2018. Students' overall rates of tobacco use rose during this period, however, due to an explosion in the popularity of electronic cigarettes. The percentage of high-school students who reported vaping in the past 30 days grew from 1.5 percent in 2011 to 20.8 percent in 2018. Counting the 4.9 percent of middle-school students who reported using e-cigarettes in 2018, the number of young people defined as "current vapers" reached 3.6 million nationwide (Office on Smoking and Health 2019).

As places where teenagers gather in large numbers and spend the majority of their waking hours, schools emerged at the forefront of the youth vaping craze. Within a few years, e-cigarettes went from virtually nonexistent to ubiquitous, and enforcement of anti-tobacco policies once again ranked among the most pressing issues facing teachers and principals. "For the longest time, nobody smoked; kids weren't into that anymore," said Brad Seamer, assistant principal of a South Dakota high school. "With the vaping, kids are really into that. It's not a certain kind of kid, it's a cross-section of my school" (Blad 2018). "It's everywhere, and my school is no different," added Francis Thompson, principal of a Connecticut high school. "I think it's the next health epidemic for kids" (Blad 2018).

Preventing students from vaping in school presents unique challenges for educators because e-cigarette use is difficult to detect. Unlike combustible cigarettes, which produce strong-smelling smoke that lingers in the air, e-cigarettes produce odorless or innocuous-smelling vapor that dissipates quickly. In addition, many vaping devices have low-profile designs that can easily be mistaken for ordinary items students might take to school, such as pens, markers, lip balm, or USB drives. The market-leading Juul brand e-cigarette, which gained so much popularity that teenagers routinely refer to vaping as "Juuling," is compact enough to fit in a pocket or be concealed in the palm of a hand. E-liquids come in many sweet flavors that appeal to young people, and some vape pods are packaged to resemble popular candy brands, such as Jolly Ranchers or Blow Pops.

Since vaping is easy to conceal, many students bring e-cigarettes to school and use them on buses, at lockers, in bathrooms, and even during class. "They can pin them onto their shirt collar or bra strap and lean over and take a hit every now and then, and who's to know?" said Howard Colter, superintendent of a Maine school district (Zernike 2018). Students share tips on social media about how to hide e-cigarettes from parents and use them at school without detection. One company, VaprWear, produces apparel and backpacks with integrated pockets to hold e-cigarettes and facilitate discreet vaping. "[Students] are very daring when it comes to [vaping in school]," said Michigan health educator Cheryl Phillips, "because it is very inconspicuous and easy to take a hit off your vape and blow the vapor into your jacket or shirt and nobody knows that you've done it" (Higgins 2018).

Growing Concerns about Student Vaping

As part of the struggle to contain student vaping, educators have sought to understand why teenagers seem to find e-cigarettes so alluring. Some point to advertising for e-cigarettes—which is not subject to the same federal regulations as cigarette advertising—for making vaping seem cool, exciting, and sexy. Others trace the popularity of vaping to social media, where trend-setting celebrities pose with vape pens in Instagram photos, hipsters demonstrate vapor tricks in YouTube videos, and millions of enthusiasts tweet their vaping experiences using such hashtags as #VapeLife or #DoIt4Juul. While some students began vaping to be cool or fit in, others did it as a form of adolescent rebellion. "It's our demon," said Nate Carpenter, vice principal of a Maine middle school. "It's the one risky thing that you can do in your life—with little consequence, in their mind—to show that you're a little bit of a rebel" (Zernike 2018).

Many students decide to experiment with vaping because they perceive e-cigarettes as harmless. "I get the sense that students think it's safe," said Cam Traut, a nurse at an Illinois high school. "The marketing or advertising was, 'oh, this is a much healthier version of traditional, tobacco cigarettes,' so the kids have focused on that 'healthier' component" (Flannery 2018). Although public health experts generally consider e-cigarettes less harmful than combustible cigarettes, they stress that the long-term health effects remain unknown. "You're not going to hear me say this thing is exactly like a cigarette. It's not," said Dave Dobbins of the Truth Initiative antismoking organization. "But there are a lot of concerns about it" (Blad 2018).

Health experts worry about the chemical additives used in e-liquids, some of which have been found to be toxic. "With cigarettes, we've been studying them for many years, we have a pretty good idea of what the risks are," said pediatric medical researcher Mark L. Rubenstein. "We just don't know what the risks of inhaling all these flavorings and dyes are, and what we do know is already pretty scary" (Zernike 2018). In one study, for instance, Rubenstein found higher levels of several carcinogenic chemicals in the urine of teenagers who used e-cigarettes than in nonusers.

Another concern is that e-cigarettes deliver nicotine, the chemical stimulant found in tobacco, which can be habit-forming or addictive. A single Juul pod contains about as much nicotine as a pack of traditional cigarettes. Yet a survey conducted by the Truth Initiative revealed that 63 percent of current vapers between the ages of 15 and 24 were not aware that e-liquids contained nicotine. "Kids don't understand what's in it," said Texas physical education teacher Valerie Phillips. "They think it's just flavored water vapor" (Korbey 2018).

Research has also shown that adolescent brains are more susceptible to nicotine addiction than adult brains. Some schools have moved away from punishing students who are repeatedly caught vaping because the students may be experiencing intense physical cravings for nicotine. "Despite all of the boundaries set by families and parents and the schools, and at risk of even expulsion, students are continuing to use," said Liz Blackwell, a school nurse in Colorado. "They don't want to be kicked out of school, they don't want to suffer any punishment or discipline, and they don't want to have a bad relationship with their parents. They continue to use because it's an addiction" (Zernike 2018).

Because early exposure to nicotine causes permanent changes in the developing adolescent brain, some researchers assert that students who use e-cigarettes may be more likely to smoke cigarettes in the future. They claim that vaping opens a gateway to smoking for teenagers who would not otherwise have tried cigarettes, thus reversing the progress of anti-smoking campaigns and creating a new generation of nicotine-dependent customers for the tobacco industry. "I have the same conversation with every student we catch vaping," said Scott Carpenter, dean of a Rhode Island high school. "I say, 'If I handed you a cigarette would you smoke it?' And 100 percent of them look at you like you're absolutely crazy for even suggesting that they'd do that" (Zernike 2018).

School Responses to Student Vaping

Student vaping has emerged as one of the most pressing disciplinary issues for school administrators. Most schools maintain tobacco-free campuses and enforce zero-tolerance policies for tobacco use, and an increasing number have updated these rules to encompass e-cigarettes and vaping. Penalties for students caught vaping include detention, suspension, and expulsion. Since e-cigarettes can be used to inhale marijuana vapor, some school districts require students in possession of vaping equipment to undergo mandatory drug testing. Recognizing the addictive capacity of nicotine, some schools focus on intervention rather than punishment. Repeat offenders may be required to meet with a counselor, attend tobacco-prevention classes, receive cessation assistance, or undergo substance-abuse treatment. "Teachers will tell you they literally have kids who can't sit through a class because they have such a strong craving for Juul," said Truth Initiative president Robin Koval. "You now have an entire population of kids who are addicted to nicotine, and we have to help them quit" (Pitofsky 2018).

Although student vaping occurs in many places on school grounds, enforcement efforts have focused mainly on bathrooms. Bathrooms have become the preferred location for vaping because they offer students privacy, freedom from security cameras, and a legitimate-seeming excuse to gather in groups. Many schools have responded to the prevalence of student vaping in bathrooms by eliminating access to some bathrooms, removing outer doors, stationing staff members in bathrooms during lunch hours and between class periods, tracking students' bathroom use throughout the day, or installing vapor detectors. Others have asked students to inform staff members if they notice multiple people in a stall or smell a fruity aroma.

Many schools have concentrated their resources on educational programs designed to prevent young people from trying e-cigarettes. A major component of these programs involves educating parents about the prevalence of vaping in school, because they are often unaware of the problem. "Over and over, we heard that the first time a parent heard about [vaping] was when they got a call from school that their student was being suspended because they were found with paraphernalia," said Cheryl Phillips (Higgins 2018). School administrators send e-mails and letters home or hold informational meetings at school to familiarize parents with e-cigarettes and help them recognize the signs that their students may be vaping.

For students, prevention programs often include presentations about the health risks associated with vaping and the addictive capacity of nicotine. The nonprofit organization CATCH My Breath offers a free, online curriculum for middle- and high-school students that identifies the potentially harmful chemicals in e-liquids and dispels the misconception that vaping is harmless fun. Other programs give students tools to help them make informed, healthy decisions about vaping. "They're learning how to deal with social pressure, how to respond to family dynamics and stress," said Ryan Crowdis, who runs a tobacco-prevention program in California (Korbey 2018).

Some schools have found peer-to-peer approaches effective in vaping prevention. In this model, high-school students complete projects on the health risks of vaping, develop anti-vaping campaigns, and share their findings with fellow students through posters, presentations, morning announcements, or assemblies. Some districts use older students as anti-vaping ambassadors, sending them to middle schools to influence younger students not to experiment with e-cigarettes. "I'm hoping that when the middle schoolers see this kid they looked up to on the basketball team saying, 'Vaping is bad for you and here's why you shouldn't do this,' it might have more impact on them than the teachers or parents saying it," said Gregg Wieczorek, a principal who implemented such a program at his Wisconsin high school (Korbey 2018).

Finally, many educators have become vocal advocates of stronger government regulation of the e-cigarette industry to reduce students' access to tobacco products. National teachers' associations have urged the U.S. Food and Drug Administration (FDA) to subject e-cigarettes to the same restrictions on advertising and sales that apply to traditional cigarettes, arguing that these measures have proven effective in reducing smoking rates among teenagers. School administrators have also expressed support for raising the federal minimum age for tobacco purchases to 21 nationwide, and for banning flavored e-liquids that appeal to young people. Some educators questioned whether any of these measures would eliminate the problem of youth vaping. "I think this is something that will remain in the fabric of adolescence," said Massachusetts high school principal Aaron Sicotte. "The access is too easy, the draw is too great, and the push through advertising is too significant" (Ibarra 2018).

In response to growing concerns about vaping in schools, Juul and other e-cigarette manufacturers have developed their own programs to prevent youth vaping. Juul announced a $30 million initiative that included an educational curriculum, improved age-verification for online sales, and the removal of flavored e-liquids from retail outlets. "We want to be a leader in seeking solutions," said Juul executive Ashley Gould, "and are actively engaged with, and listening to, community leaders, educators, and lawmakers on how best to effectively keep young people away from Juul" (Blad 2018). Supporters of vaping as a reduced-harm alternative to combustible cigarettes worried that some of these measures would restrict the choices available to adult smokers who were trying to quit. They urged the FDA and e-cigarette producers not to overreact to reports of youth vaping, which they described as normal adolescent experimentation. Vaping supporters also claimed that e-cigarettes posed fewer health risks than many common teen risk behaviors, including cigarette smoking.

Further Reading

Blad, Evie. 2018. "'Juuling' Craze: Schools Struggle to Deal with Student Vaping." *Education Week* 37 (30): 1, May 4, 2018. https://www.edweek.org/ew/arti cles/2018/05/09/juuling-craze-schools-scramble-to-deal-with.html.

Flannery, Mary Ellen. 2018. "Vaping in Schools: 3 Million Students and Counting." NEA Today, November 14, 2018. http://neatoday.org/2018/11/14 /vaping-in-schools/.

Higgins, Lori. 2018. "Your Kids Think It's Cool to Vape at School. It's a Big Problem." *Detroit Free Press*, September 25, 2018. https://www.freep.com /story/news/education/2018/09/25/vaping-teens-school/1404821002/.

Ibarra, Anna B. 2018. "Why Juuling Has Become a Nightmare for School Administrators." NBC News, March 26, 2018. https://www.nbcnews.com/health

/kids-health/why-juuling-has-become-nightmare-school-administrators
-n860106.

Korbey, Holly. 2018. "Schools Respond to the Rise of Student Vaping." Edutopia,
June 29, 2018. https://www.edutopia.org/article/schools-respond-rise
-student-vaping.

Office on Smoking and Health. 2019. "Youth and Tobacco Use." U.S. Centers for
Disease Control and Prevention, February 5, 2019. https://www.cdc.gov
/tobacco/data_statistics/fact_sheets/youth_data/tobacco_use/index.htm.

Pitofsky, Marina. 2018. "Millions of Teens Are Vaping Every Day. Here's What
They Have to Say about the Growing Trend." *USA Today*, December 20,
2018. https://www.usatoday.com/story/news/2018/12/20/teen-vaping
-rise-here-why/2239155002/.

Zernike, Kate. 2018. "'I Can't Stop': Schools Struggle with Vaping Explosion."
New York Times, April 2, 2018. https://www.nytimes.com/2018/04/02
/health/vaping-ecigarettes-addiction-teen.html.

Vaping and Youth Culture

From the rugged Marlboro Man cowboy to the popular cartoon character Joe Camel, classic cigarette advertising often projected an image of smoking as exciting, cool, and rebellious. The tobacco companies also added appealing flavors to their products to reduce the harshness, improve the taste, and help initiate new smokers. Antismoking activists charged that these tactics were intended to convince young people to try cigarettes. Since the developing adolescent brain is highly susceptible to the addictive effects of nicotine, attracting young people to cigarettes increased the tobacco industry's chances of gaining long-term customers. Studies have shown that 90 percent of adult smokers tried their first cigarette before age 18, while only 1 percent began smoking after age 26. "Smoking initiation is an adolescent thing," said tobacco industry researcher Robert Jackler. "They smoke, they get hooked on the nicotine, and they become lifelong consumers" (Keller 2018).

Antismoking advocates credit federal regulations on cigarette advertising and tobacco flavoring for helping to reduce the appeal of smoking to young people. Along with successful tobacco-control campaigns that raised public awareness of the health risks associated with cigarettes and secondhand smoke, these measures changed teenagers' attitudes about smoking and led to a dramatic decline in youth smoking rates. Following the introduction of electronic cigarettes, however, the downward trend in adolescent tobacco use suddenly reversed. Especially after the Juul brand came on the market in 2015, youth vaping exploded in popularity. "It's kind of like its own culture at this point," said Leia Dyste, an undergraduate student at Northern Arizona University. "I think a lot of people feel left out if they don't have a vape to just pull out at any time" (Pitofsky 2018).

Critics noted that e-cigarettes were not subject to the same restrictions on advertising and flavoring that applied to conventional tobacco products. They argued that e-cigarette manufacturers—which were increasingly affiliated with the big tobacco companies—adopted many of the same youth-oriented marketing strategies that had been used to sell cigarettes, including colorful advertising campaigns and sweet, fruity flavors. In addition, e-cigarette producers took full advantage of social media to shape teens' perceptions of vaping, promoting it as fun, glamourous, edgy, and cool. "They do the same damn thing today as they did then," Jackler said of e-cigarette marketing. "The messaging is very subtle, very carefully crafted. They target, in the same way, adolescents" (Keller 2018). Alarmed by the rapid increase in youth vaping, public health officials sought ways to counteract the influence of social media and reduce the impact of e-cigarettes on teen health and culture.

E-Cigarette Advertisements Proliferate

Cigarette advertisements have been banned from U.S. radio and television since 1971, and from billboards, public transit, and event sponsorship since 1998. The Family Smoking Prevention and Tobacco Control Act of 2009 enacted further restrictions against cigarette marketing strategies that targeted children. As a result, a generation of Americans largely escaped the influence of messages promoting tobacco products. When the first e-cigarettes appeared in the United States in 2007, however, they were not subject to the same advertising restrictions as combustible cigarettes. Operating in an environment that Jackler described as an "unregulated Wild West" (Keller 2018), e-cigarette manufacturers adopted some of the same marketing approaches that had proven successful for tobacco companies in the past.

Advertising for vaping products—which Jackler called "manifestly youth-oriented" (Nedelman, Selig, and Azad 2019)—featured bright colors and geometric shapes, attractive young models, celebrity endorsements, cartoon characters, and themes of freedom, independence, and elevated social status. E-cigarette producers sponsored film festivals and sporting events and gave away free samples at concerts, nightclubs, and cultural events. Some companies offered college scholarships in exchange for essays promoting the benefits of vaping. Many e-cigarette ads portrayed vaping as harmless fun and minimized the risk of nicotine addiction. "It's the only source of information that most consumers have about e-cigarettes, and they're portraying them as safe and healthy alternatives," said public health researcher Jennifer Duke. "They're glamorized in these advertisements as modern and a fun adult activity. So I don't think it's surprising that youth also find these products appealing" (Pearson 2015).

E-cigarette advertisements appeared in many sources that banned traditional cigarette advertisements, such as television and billboards, and they reached a broad audience that included underage youth. The U.S. Centers for Disease Control and Prevention (CDC) found that four out of five middle-school and high-school students—or 20.5 million kids nationwide—were exposed to e-cigarette ads from at least one source in 2016. Retail stores accounted for the largest share of youth exposure, followed by the Internet, television and movies, and print media (Simon 2018).

Studies suggest that young people who are exposed to e-cigarette promotions are more likely to experiment with vaping. A survey of 7,000 teenagers who had never used tobacco products, for instance, found that respondents who remembered seeing e-cigarette ads were 1.6 times more interested in trying the products than those who had not seen the ads (Keller 2018). "No one was really into [vaping] until the Juuls came out," said James McCall, an undergraduate student at James Madison University. "They definitely had ads in the past that had teenage-looking people in the ad, and it had lots of moving around and catchy music. Whoever was viewing it definitely got a party vibe" (Pitofsky 2018).

Critics charged that e-cigarette manufacturers intentionally targeted young people in their advertising, as the tobacco industry had done in the past, in order to create a new generation of nicotine users. They called for strict federal regulation of e-cigarette marketing as part of a youth tobacco-prevention initiative. "These ads are designed to appeal to users who are not of age," wrote the authors of a Stanford University study of e-cigarette advertisements. "There definitely are a lot of consequences socially with that. E-cigarette companies have a bigger role to play in terms of being more responsible citizens" (Keller 2018).

Juul and other e-cigarette companies claimed that antismoking activists mischaracterized their marketing messages. They insisted that vaping products were designed as a reduced-harm alternative for adult cigarette smokers, and they argued that their goal was to disrupt the tobacco industry rather than emulate it. "It is absolutely false that Juul markets to anyone other than adult smokers," a Juul representative said in a statement. "No young person, and no adult who is already not a smoker, should use our product or any nicotine product. All of our marketing reflects that position" (Keller 2018). As Juul's popularity among teenagers brought its marketing tactics under scrutiny by the U.S. Food and Drug Administration (FDA), however, the company acknowledged that its initial advertising campaign inadvertently appealed to young people. "That campaign in the end, we felt, did not help us achieve our mission of speaking to adult smokers to provide them information about an alternative to cigarettes," said Juul executive Ashley Gould (Nedelman, Selig, and Azad 2019).

Advocates of vaping oppose most restrictions on e-cigarette advertising, arguing that Juul and other manufacturers should be allowed to build brand recognition, promote technological innovations, and communicate the reduced-harm benefits of their products to smokers. They contend that excessive regulation of e-cigarette marketing is counterproductive to public health goals because it protects the big tobacco companies from competition and places more lives at risk from smoking-related diseases. They propose a limited regulatory scheme for e-cigarette advertising that prohibits the inclusion of misleading statements and themes intended to appeal to underage youth.

Vaping Goes Viral on Social Media

Juul took advantage of the viral power of social media to spread the word about its products. The company's 2015 launch campaign, "Vaporized," was powered by marketing pushes on various social media platforms, including Twitter, Instagram, and YouTube. The content of the advertisements initiated by Juul featured sexy models in their twenties relaxing, having fun, or partying with a Juul. "What Juul did that's different is it exploited social media, where American middle and high school kids live," Jackler explained. "That was their innovation" (Belluz 2019).

During its initial campaign, Juul also paid several social media influencers to promote its products to their followers using such hashtags as #juul, #vaporized, #juulvapor, #switchtojuul, and #doit4juul. Although the company claimed that it hired only influencers who were former cigarette smokers over the age of 28, the campaigns spread quickly to a wide audience online. "Social media works differently than other stuff. You don't need that many people," said Matthew L. Myers, president of the Campaign for Tobacco-Free Kids. "A small number of people who are popular and get reposted can reach a very large number of people" (Nedelman, Selig, and Azad 2018).

Social media users soon began creating and posting their own Juul-related content, including memes, images, tricks involving clouds of vapor, and tips for vaping discreetly in public. "You started seeing viral peer-to-peer communication among teens who basically became brand ambassadors for Juul," Jackler noted (Brodwin 2018). Juul engaged with social media users by offering discounts, commenting on posts, and reposting photos of Juul products in use. In a representative 2017 tweet, which featured an image of a Juul device next to a dessert, the company encouraged its followers on Twitter to "RT if you enjoy dessert without the spoon with our Crème Brulée #juulpods" (Pitofsky 2018). Although Juul executives claimed that they did not intend to target underage people, Jackler asserted that "their way of promoting their product had great appeal to young people and caused a market fervor" (Nedelman, Selig, and Azad 2018). One study estimated that people under age 18 accounted for one-fourth of Juul's Twitter followers (Chu et al 2018).

As Juul gained traction on social media, its sales increased dramatically. From 2015 to 2017, according to one study, the average number of Juul-related tweets on Twitter grew from 765 per month to 30,565 per month. Over that same period, the seven Instagram sites that posted the most Juul-related content amassed more than 250,000 followers. Juul's viral presence on social media helped it go from a little-known company to the leader of the vaping industry, capturing more than half of the U.S. market by 2018 (Huang 2018). After Juul's initial marketing push, most of the millions of Juul-related photos, videos, memes, and blog posts on social media were generated by users of the device—some of them teenagers—who were not affiliated with the company. Although Juul did not create the content, it helped make vaping part of youth culture. "What resonates with our generation *is* the memes," Connecticut high-school student Brennan McDermott told the *New York Times*. "You'll see a bunch of memes about Juuling. It's just, like, making it more socially acceptable—it's perpetuating the thing that vaping is cool" (Barshad 2018).

As rates of youth vaping increased, tobacco-control advocates demanded that the FDA crack down on the marketing practices used by Juul and other e-cigarette manufacturers. "This will only be stemmed with really strong action by the FDA," Myers stated. "The FDA has the authority to say to JUUL that they have to prove that it helps smokers quit, it does not appeal to kids, and that flavors don't appeal to kids—and the FDA can pull the product [off the market]" (Zimlich 2018). While the FDA had the authority to regulate e-cigarette advertising, however, its options were limited when it came to controlling social media posts by vaping enthusiasts.

As Juul increasingly came under scrutiny by federal regulators for its role in precipitating a youth vaping "epidemic," the company made a number of moves intended to reduce underage exposure and access to its products. Juul Labs deleted its Facebook and Instagram profiles, limited its use of Twitter to non-promotional messages, and established an internal team to identify and report inappropriate third-party social media content. Juul also shifted its advertising strategy to focus on testimonials by adult cigarette smokers who experienced health benefits by switching to Juul. Critics argued that the company's response did little to resolve the problem. "Although Juul is taking measures now to address the virality of its products among teenagers, it's too little, too late," Jackler said (Brodwin 2018). "The Juul hashtag lives on," he added. "It's immortal. It's still viral in peer-to-peer teen promotion" (Belluz 2019).

Flavored E-Liquids Appeal to Youth

Some critics attribute the popularity of vaping among teenagers to the availability and appeal of flavored e-liquids. The tobacco industry had a long history of adding flavor to cigarettes, cigars, and other tobacco products to reduce the harshness, improve the taste, and attract new customers. Public health officials recognized that flavored tobacco products held a strong appeal for young people, who tended to perceive them as less harmful and more fun than ordinary tobacco products. The Family Smoking Prevention and Tobacco Control Act of 2009 sought to address this problem by banning the use of flavors in cigarettes except for menthol, a minty flavor that creates a cooling sensation to counteract the heat in inhaled smoke. The law did not restrict the use of flavors in tobacco products other than cigarettes, however, and e-cigarette manufacturers took advantage of the loophole. "The tobacco industry knows that mint and menthol help the poison go down," said Erika Sward of the American Lung Association. "And they have been using menthol cigarettes to addict millions of people for decades, and that trend has tragically continued with e-cigarettes" (Reinberg 2018).

E-cigarette companies developed and marketed e-liquids in thousands of different flavors. Tobacco-control advocates assert that the sweet and fruity flavors—such as birthday cake, cotton candy, s'mores, cookies and cream, gummi bear, and cherry cola—seem designed to entice underage youth to experiment with vaping. In addition, the wide assortment of flavors seems intended to promote continued use, as young people indulge their curiosity or sense of novelty by trying out appealing new flavors and trading with their friends. Many flavored e-liquids come in packaging designed to resemble snack foods and beverages that are popular with children, such as juice boxes, candy, or cookies.

Research has shown that flavors play an important role in youth tobacco use. One study found that 81 percent of underage tobacco users started out with a flavored product (Rapaport 2019). In a 2018 study, 78 percent of teenage vapers cited appealing flavors as a major factor in their decision to use e-cigarettes (Becker 2019). "If flavors aren't the No. 1 reason teens are using Juul, they're No. 2," Koval said. "Flavors use the same reasoning that kids are using when they're in a candy store" (Pitofsky 2018).

Responding to growing concerns about the prevalence of youth vaping, the FDA took steps to reduce the appeal and availability of flavored tobacco products in 2018. The agency cracked down on companies that used deceptive packaging to make e-liquids look like kid-friendly foods, for instance, and proposed a ban on the sale of flavored tobacco products at ordinary retail outlets, such as convenience stores and gas stations. Under the FDA rule, flavored e-liquids could be sold only through vape shops and other outlets with age-restricted access or through Internet sites equipped with age-verification technology. Then-FDA Commissioner Scott Gottlieb said that the measures aimed "to strike a careful public health balance between our imperative to enable the opportunities to transition to non-combustible products to be available for adults and our solemn mandate to make nicotine products less accessible and less appealing to children" (Haelle 2018).

Many adults who switched to e-cigarettes as a reduced-harm alternative to combustible cigarettes objected to the flavor restrictions, arguing that flavored e-liquids were enjoyable and helped them quit smoking. Some vaping supporters claimed that limiting access for underage youth also limited the options available to adults who relied on e-cigarettes as smoking-cessation tools. "Not every town has a vape shop," said Greg Conley, president of the American Vaping Association. "For many adults, it will be much easier to pick up a pack of Marlboros or Camels—or even an unrestricted cherry-flavored cigar—at a local convenience store than it will be to make the switch to a vaping product that can truly help smokers break their desire for cigarettes" (Haelle 2018).

Tobacco-control advocates, in turn, called for an outright federal ban on flavored tobacco products. They cited research suggesting teenagers were three to four times more likely to vape fruit-flavored or candy-flavored e-liquids than adults (Becker 2019). "Even with new sales restrictions announced today by FDA preventing flavored e-cigarettes from being sold at certain brick and mortar storefronts, teens will still find ways to access them," said Colleen Kraft, president of the American Academy of Pediatrics. "E-cigarette products that appeal to children have no business in the marketplace, period. FDA must take stronger action to protect young people" (Haelle 2018).

Further Reading

Barshad, Amos. 2018. "The Juul Is Too Cool." *New York Times*, April 7, 2018. https://www.nytimes.com/2018/04/07/style/the-juul-is-too-cool.html.

Becker, Rachel. 2019. "Flavored Vapes Draw FDA Ire, with Some Exceptions." The Verge, March 13, 2019. https://www.theverge.com/2019/3/13/18264 575/fda-electronic-cigarettes-flavorings-vaping-nicotine-mint-menthol.

Belluz, Julia. 2019. "The Vape Company Juul Said It Doesn't Target Teens. It's Early Ads Tell a Different Story." Vox, January 25, 2019. https://www.vox .com/2019/1/25/18194953/vape-juul-e-cigarette-marketing.

Brodwin, Erin. 2018. "See How Juul Turned Teens into Influencers and Threw Buzzy Parties to Fuel Its Rise as Silicon Valley's Favorite E-Cig Company." Business Insider, November 26, 2018. https://www.businessin sider.com/stanford-juul-ads-photos-teens-e-cig-vaping-2018-11.

Chu, Kar-Hai, et al. 2018. "Juul: Spreading Online and Offline." *Journal of Adolescent Health* 63 (5): 582, November 2018. https://www.jahonline.org/article /S1054-139X(18)30358-6/fulltext.

Gross, Liza. 2017. "Smoke Screen." The Verge, November 16, 2017. https://www .theverge.com/2017/11/16/16658358/vape-lobby-vaping-health-risks -nicotine-big-tobacco-marketing.

Haelle, Tara. 2018. "FDA Ban on E-Cigarette Flavors: A Showdown between Protecting Kids and Reducing Harm." *Forbes*, November 15, 2018. https:// www.forbes.com/sites/tarahaelle/2018/11/15/fda-ban-on-e-cigarette -flavors-a-showdown-between-protecting-kids-and-reducing-harm /#22e67b441b68.

Huang, Jidong, et al. 2018. "Vaping versus JUULing: How the Extraordinary Growth and Marketing of JUUL Transformed the US Retail E-Cigarette Market." *Tobacco Control*, May 31, 2018. https://tobaccocontrol.bmj.com/content /tobaccocontrol/early/2018/05/31/tobaccocontrol-2018-054382.full.pdf.

Keller, Kate. 2018. "Ads for E-Cigarettes Today Hearken Back to the Banned Tricks of Big Tobacco." *Smithsonian*, April 11, 2018. https://www.smithso nianmag.com/history/electronic-cigarettes-millennial-appeal-ushers -next-generation-nicotine-addicts-180968747/#37DvuPF0vSVtK3i9.99.

Nedelman, Michael, Roni Selig, and Arman Azad. 2018. "#JUUL: How Social Media Hyped Nicotine for a New Generation." CNN, December 19, 2018. https://www.cnn.com/2018/12/17/health/juul-social-media-influencers /index.html.

Pearson, Carol. 2015. "Report: E-Cigarettes Can Cause Permanent Brain Damage for Teens." Voice of America, April 30, 2015. https://www.voanews .com/a/report-e-cigarettes-can-cause-permanent-brain-damage-for -teens/2744206.html.

Pitofsky, Marina. 2018. "Millions of Teens Are Vaping Every Day. Here's What They Have to Say about the Growing Trend." *USA Today*, December 20, 2018. https://www.usatoday.com/story/news/2018/12/20/teen-vaping -rise-here-why/2239155002/.

Rapaport, Lisa. 2019. "Flavored Tobacco Use Rising in U.S. Kids as Vaping Takes Off." Reuters, January 7, 2019. https://www.reuters.com/article/us-health -teens-smoking/flavored-tobacco-use-rising-in-us-kids-as-vaping-takes -off-idUSKCN1P129X.

Reinberg, Steven. 2018. "1 in 5 U.S. High School Students Now Vapes: CDC." HealthDay, November 15, 2018. https://consumer.healthday.com/cancer -information-5/electronic-cigarettes-970/1-in-5-u-s-high-school-students -now-vapes-cdc-739733.html.

Simon, Stacy. 2018. "Report: More and More Teens Seeing E-Cigarette Ads." American Cancer Society, March 19, 2018. https://www.cancer.org /latest-news/report-more-and-more-teens-seeing-e-cigarette-ads.html.

Zimlich, Rachael. 2018. "How Tobacco and Vaping Marketing Is Changing." *Contemporary Pediatrics*, October 3, 2018. https://www.contemporarype diatrics.com/pediatrics/how-tobacco-and-vaping-marketing-changing.

E-Cigarettes and Global Health Policy

More than 40 million people around the world used e-cigarettes in 2018, up from around 7 million in 2011, and the market for vaping products reached $22 billion worldwide. The United States accounted for the largest share of global e-cigarette sales, followed by Japan and the United Kingdom (Jones 2018). By comparison, the number of cigarette smokers around the world reached 1.12 billion in 2018. The countries of Eastern and Central Europe ranked highest in annual cigarette consumption per capita, while the United States ranked 68th globally (Smith 2018).

The World Health Organization (WHO) considers cigarette smoking a major threat to global health. More than 7 million people died from smoking-related diseases or exposure to secondhand smoke in 2018, at an estimated economic cost to society of $2 trillion (Smith 2018). The WHO helps United Nations member-states develop policies to reduce rates of tobacco use and prevent smoking-related diseases and premature deaths. The WHO's main antismoking tool is the Framework Convention on Tobacco Control (FCTC), a landmark treaty that established global standards intended to "protect present and future generations from the devastating health, social, environmental, and economic consequences of tobacco consumption and exposure to tobacco smoke" (WHO FCTC 2003).

Electronic cigarettes became available internationally shortly after the FCTC took effect in 2005. Some e-cigarette manufacturers marketed their products as healthier forms of nicotine delivery that could help tobacco users alleviate the desire to smoke. Vaping proponents claimed that e-cigarettes advanced the WHO's overall goal of reducing the harmful health effects of tobacco consumption. As health claims associated with e-cigarettes proliferated, however, public health experts grew concerned that millions of people were adopting the new technology before it had been adequately tested. In 2008, WHO officials issued a formal statement warning individuals and governments that the alleged benefits of vaping remained unproven. The WHO warning about e-cigarettes convinced several FCTC signatory nations to ban the devices—including Australia, Brazil, Canada, Hong Kong, Panama, and Saudi Arabia—while dozens of other countries scrambled to enact regulations on e-cigarette production, marketing, sale, and usage.

WHO's Cautious Stance Ignites Controversy

Over the next few years, WHO scientists conducted research on the effects of e-cigarettes and reviewed evidence from around the world. They used this information to develop a set of policy recommendations for FCTC countries regarding e-cigarettes. In a report published in 2013, the WHO Tobacco Free Initiative urged governments to subject vaping products to many of the same regulations as conventional cigarettes. The recommendations included developing standards for product safety, establishing minimum-age restrictions for sales, prohibiting the use of sweet flavors that might appeal to children, banning vaping in public places, restricting advertising media and content, and prohibiting e-cigarette manufacturers from making health claims without evidence.

Vaping advocates criticized the WHO's cautious approach toward e-cigarette regulation, claiming that it overstated the health risks of e-cigarettes and underestimated their potential as a reduced-harm alternative to combustible cigarettes. Critics argued that the WHO should encourage existing cigarette smokers to switch to e-cigarettes, which could help reduce global smoking rates and smoking-related diseases. In 2014, a group of 53 prominent public health experts from around the world published a letter asking the WHO to reconsider its stance on vaping. "These products could be among the most significant health innovations of the 21st century—perhaps saving hundreds of millions of lives," they wrote. "We are deeply concerned that the classification of these products as tobacco and their inclusion in the FCTC will do more harm than good. . . . We hope that under your leadership, the WHO and FCTC will be in the vanguard of science-based, effective, and ethical tobacco policy, embracing tobacco harm reduction" (Abrams et al 2014).

Although WHO leaders acknowledged that vaping appeared to be safer than smoking, they continued to insist that further research was needed to prove its health benefits. "Average e-cigarettes are likely to be less toxic than conventional cigarettes, although they are not without risks," said WHO tobacco-control expert Armando Peruga. "Some people say these risks are very, very low, but our question is 'how low?' If smoking a cigarette is like jumping from the 100th floor, using an e-cigarette is certainly like jumping from a lower floor, but which floor? We don't know" (Fleck 2014). WHO scientists expressed concern about the addictive capacity of nicotine in e-liquids and the potential health risks associated with inhaling toxic chemicals in e-cigarette vapor. They also worried about the potential for young people to experiment with vaping, become hooked on nicotine, and eventually progress to smoking combustible cigarettes.

The WHO used such concerns to justify recommending broad restrictions on e-cigarettes in UN member-states. The expressed goals for national-level regulation included deterring nonsmokers and young people from trying e-cigarettes, minimizing the potential health risks of vaping for both users and bystanders, preventing manufacturers from making unsubstantiated health and safety claims, and barring tobacco-industry involvement in e-cigarette advertising. "The main disagreement is over what to do in terms of regulation and what regulation can achieve, given that current scientific evidence on e-cigarettes is limited," Peruga said of the strong opposition from vaping advocates. "Our view is that regulation should bring the best out of any product while minimizing the worst: a very difficult balance to achieve" (Fleck 2014).

Approaches to E-Cigarette Regulation around the World

Regulation of e-cigarettes varies widely between nations. According to the Institute for Global Tobacco Control, 98 countries had national laws regulating the product design, manufacturing, packaging, distribution, marketing, sale, or use of e-cigarettes as of 2018. While some countries wrote new regulations to apply specifically to e-cigarettes, others subjected vaping products to tobacco-control policies already in place. The WHO FCTC served as the basis for many of the government policies regarding vaping products.

Twenty-nine countries banned the sale of e-cigarettes entirely, while other countries subjected them to regulation as tobacco products, medical devices, consumer products, hazardous substances, or vaping products.

Like the United States, which set the federal age to purchase vaping products at 18, 36 countries established a minimum legal age for e-cigarette sales between 16 and 21. Sixty-seven countries, including the United States, regulated or prohibited advertising and promotion of vaping products. In terms of e-cigarette packaging, 31 countries required child-safety standards and 38 countries required printed health warning labels, including the United States. Many national regulations concern the content of e-liquids, with 32 countries limiting the concentration of nicotine, 32 prohibiting the use of toxic ingredients, and 31 controlling product quality or flavoring. A total of 51 countries had policies prohibiting vaping in public places, while 13 countries subjected e-cigarettes to taxation (Institute for Global Tobacco Control 2018).

Australia and Canada are among the nations that created a de facto ban on e-cigarettes by defining nicotine as a drug or poison and making it illegal to sell without government approval. In both cases, however, e-cigarettes still became widely available online or through black-market supply channels. A 2016 study found that 49 percent of cigarette smokers in Canada and 45 percent of smokers in Australia had tried vaping, with 5.5 percent in Canada and 6 percent in Australia defining themselves as current e-cigarette users (Gravely 2018). Vaping supporters in both countries called on the national governments to loosen restrictions on e-cigarettes and promote vaping as a reduced-harm alternative to cigarettes. Citing concerns about potential health risks and youth vaping, Australia maintained a strict regulatory approach consistent with the FCTC, requiring users to obtain a prescription for e-liquids containing nicotine. In 2018, Canada passed the Tobacco and Vaping Products Act, which legalized the sale of e-cigarettes as reduced-harm alternatives for adult smokers while also restricting youth access to nicotine-containing products.

The European Union adopted a regulatory approach that defines e-cigarettes as tobacco products and subjects them to many of the same restrictions that apply to cigarettes. Under the Tobacco Products Directive, enacted in 2016, all e-liquids sold in the 28 EU member-states were required to have a nicotine concentration lower than 20 mg/mL. Vaping supporters criticized this measure as arbitrary and argued that it limited the effectiveness of e-cigarettes as smoking-cessation tools. The EU directive also banned most e-cigarette advertising, promotion, and sponsorship and required vaping product packaging to include health warnings, complete lists of ingredients, and information about toxicity and addiction. Despite such restrictions, a 2017 survey showed that 15 percent of EU residents had tried vaping (Glantz 2018).

The United Kingdom, in contrast, adopted a progressive approach that promotes e-cigarette use as a form of tobacco harm reduction. As early as 2015, Public Health England released a report that declared vaping to be 95 percent safer than smoking cigarettes (Public Health England 2018). Vaping is allowed in most public places in England, with the exception of mass transit, and most regulations aim to ensure product quality and consumer safety. Like EU countries, though, the UK places limits on the nicotine concentration in e-liquids as well as the size of e-liquid containers.

In general, research suggests that rates of e-cigarette awareness, trial, and usage in countries around the world correlate more strongly with national income levels than with the extent of regulation. Vaping rates tend to be higher in high-income countries and lower in low-income countries, regardless of the government restrictions placed upon e-cigarette marketing, sale, and usage. A study of 13 countries participating in the WHO's International Tobacco Control Policy Evaluation Project (ITC Project), for instance, found 99 percent awareness of e-cigarettes among current and former cigarette smokers in four high-income countries—the United States, England, Canada, and Australia—even though the first two ranked among the "less restrictive" and the second two among the "more restrictive" in terms of national vaping laws. E-cigarette awareness was significantly lower in all of the low-income and middle-income countries, which ranged from "more restrictive" vaping laws to "no e-cigarette policies" (Gravely 2018).

Further Reading

Abrams, David, et al. 2014. "Statement from Specialists in Nicotine Science and Public Health Policy." May 26, 2014. https://nicotinepolicy.net/documents/letters/MargaretChan.pdf.

Fleck, Fiona. 2014. "Countries Vindicate Cautious Stance on E-Cigarettes." *Bulletin of the World Health Organization* 92 (12): 856, December 2014. https://www.who.int/bulletin/volumes/92/12/14-031214/en/.

Glantz, Stanton A. 2018. "European Public Health Association Releases Comprehensive, Up-to-Date Summary of the Science on E-Cigs." Center for Tobacco Control Research and Education, University of California–San Francisco, August 31, 2018. https://tobacco.ucsf.edu/european-public-health-association-releases-comprehensive-date-summary-science-e-cigs.

Gravely, Shannon, et al. 2018. "Use of Electronic Cigarettes across 13 ITC Countries with Different Regulatory Environments." *Tobacco Induced Disease* 16 (1): 229.

Institute for Global Tobacco Control. 2018. "Country Laws Regulating E-ciga-
    rettes: A Policy Scan." Baltimore: Johns Hopkins Bloomberg School of
    Public Health, November 2, 2018. https://www.globaltobaccocontrol.org
    /e-cigarette_policyscan.
Jones, Lora. 2018. "Vaping—The Rise in Five Charts." BBC News, May 31, 2018.
    https://www.bbc.com/news/business-44295336.
Kennedy, Ryan D., Ayodeji Awopegba, Elaine De León, and Joanna E. Cohen.
    2016. "Global Approaches to Regulating Electronic Cigarettes." *Tobacco
    Control* 26 (4): 440–445, November 30, 2016. https://tobaccocontrol.bmj
    .com/content/26/4/440.
Public Health England. 2018. "E-Cigarettes and Vaping: Policy, Regulation, and
    Guidance." GOV.UK, April 16, 2018. https://www.gov.uk/government
    /collections/e-cigarettes-and-vaping-policy-regulation-and-guidance.
Smith, Oliver. 2018. "Mapped: The Countries That Smoke the Most." *Telegraph*,
    May 31, 2018. https://www.telegraph.co.uk/travel/maps-and-graphics
    /world-according-to-tobacco-consumption/.
WHO Framework Convention on Tobacco Control. 2003. Geneva: World Health
    Organization.   https://apps.who.int/iris/bitstream/handle/10665/42811
    /9241591013.pdf;jsessionid=CAD8596CECD91A1B42E1F1F4FFABA231
    ?sequence=1.

E-Cigarettes and the Tobacco Industry

For decades, the tobacco industry ranked among the most powerful
and influential business enterprises in the United States. It used its financial resources and political clout to mislead the American people about
the dangers of smoking and evade government regulation of its products.
It took years of scientific research, public health campaigns, investigations, lawsuits, and tobacco-control legislation to end the deceptive practices of Big Tobacco and protect citizens from the health risks of cigarettes.
As a result of these efforts, adult cigarette smoking rates have declined
significantly from their peak of around 40 percent in the 1960s—before
the U.S. Surgeon General released the first report explicitly linking smoking to lung cancer—to reach a record low of 14 percent in 2017 (Thomas
2018).

Although antismoking campaigns and smoke-free policies contributed
to the decline in cigarette smoking, the growing popularity of vaping has
also played a role. "It's the most disruptive change in the tobacco market,"
said Jeff Drope, a health policy expert with the American Cancer Society.
"There is no parallel" (Abate 2017). Before the introduction of e-cigarettes
in 2007, cigarette sales volumes typically dropped by 3 to 4 percent per
year in the United States, and the tobacco companies compensated for the

loss of revenue by raising prices. In 2018, however, U.S. cigarette sales volumes declined by 6 percent during the first quarter alone (Gurdus 2018), and the five largest global tobacco companies lost an estimated $127 billion in market value (Mead 2018). Meanwhile, the leading e-cigarette brand, Juul, experienced 940 percent sales growth in 2018 (LaVito 2018), and experts predicted an annual growth rate in the global vaping market of over 20 percent (Mead 2018). "The tobacco industry is facing an existential threat from its vaporizer competitors, led by Juul Labs," said CNBC stock-market analyst Jim Cramer. "The cigarette industry seems to be in serious trouble" (Gurdus 2018).

Introduced in 2015, Juul quickly emerged as the dominant e-cigarette brand. The innovative device attracted consumers with its sleek, high-tech design, compact size, affordable price, ease of use, high nicotine content, and appealing flavors. Vaping enthusiasts asserted that Juul and other e-cigarettes delivered nicotine in a less harmful and more socially acceptable manner than combustible cigarettes. Many former cigarette smokers switched to vaping as a harm-reduction strategy or smoking-cessation tool, thus reducing the tobacco companies' customer base. A survey of 19,000 Juul users conducted by Juul Labs found that 62 percent had smoked cigarettes prior to trying Juul, and two-thirds of those had quit smoking after taking up vaping (Aiello 2018). "This thing is selling like crazy," Cramer said, "and it's really eating into the tobacco industry in a way that other e-cigs never could" (Gurdus 2018).

Tobacco Companies Enter the Vaping Market

In the face of growing concerns about smoking-related diseases and stricter federal regulation of tobacco products, the large cigarette manufacturers experimented with smokeless cigarettes for many years. They also introduced light, low-tar, and filtered cigarettes, which they portrayed as reduced-harm alternatives. The non-combustible products that reached market failed to catch on with consumers, however, so the tobacco companies continued to focus on their profitable existing cigarette lines. Once e-cigarettes proved to be commercially viable—especially when Juul's phenomenal popularity became clear—tobacco industry leaders recognized vaping as a potential threat to their continued viability.

Some large cigarette producers responded to the threat by investing in research and development, procuring patents, or acquiring small, independent e-cigarette producers. Lorillard Tobacco Company, one-time maker of Newport, Kent, and True cigarettes, became the first tobacco giant to expand into the vaping market by purchasing the blu e-cigarette brand in 2012 (three years later, ownership of blu shifted to the European tobacco giant Imperial Brands). R. J. Reynolds, producer of Kool, Winston, Camel, and Pall Mall cigarettes, launched its own Vuse e-cigarette line in 2013. Europe's leading tobacco company, British American Tobacco, invested $1 billion in e-cigarette development to create the Vype ePen. Altria, formerly known as Philip Morris, introduced the MarkTen e-cigarette brand in 2014.

By 2018, however, Juul controlled 75 percent of the U.S. e-cigarette market, while brands marketed by the big tobacco companies accounted for only 20 percent combined (LaVito 2018). In December of that year, Juul Labs announced a deal with Altria, manufacturer of the best-selling Marlboro cigarette brand. Altria paid $12.8 billion to acquire a 35 percent stake in Juul and subsequently discontinued production of its MarkTen e-cigarette. The high-profile collaboration generated a great deal of controversy within the vaping industry. "An industry that emerged as a potential alternative to traditional tobacco, and was once populated with smaller independent manufacturers, is now dominated by Big Tobacco," one analyst noted. "By controlling this business, Big Tobacco effectively controls its own competition" (Jain 2018).

Critics expressed misgivings about the growing involvement of major tobacco companies in the vaping industry. A survey of current adult vapers in the United States and Canada found that 73 percent held a predominantly negative opinion of e-cigarette brands owned by tobacco firms. Many of the respondents had switched to vaping from smoking and blamed the tobacco industry for encouraging their former cigarette habit (Jain 2018). Some vaping enthusiasts worried that the tobacco companies would increase e-cigarette prices, eliminate product lines, or suppress innovation in an effort to drive vapers back to smoking cigarettes, which provided higher profit margins. Some analysts predicted that vaping enthusiasts would avoid e-cigarette brands associated with large tobacco companies and instead purchase specialty products from small, independent manufacturers, such as SMOK and Vaporesso.

Other critics asserted that tobacco-company involvement in the vaping industry cast doubt on the health claims made by Juul and other e-cigarette makers. Altria executives justified their investment in Juul by saying that it reflected their mission of promoting tobacco harm reduction. Antismoking advocates questioned this claim, however, pointing out that many of the cigarette products that were marketed as reduced-harm alternatives turned out to be as bad or worse for smokers' health than regular cigarettes. They argued that the tobacco industry's long history of deceptive practices proved that its only interest was making money. "Altria largely invests in markets with a capacity for addiction, abuse, or dependency," one analyst wrote. "It doesn't invest in products with an eye toward their medical benefits" (Hiltzik 2018).

Some critics contended that the tobacco industry expanded into vaping products in an attempt to rehabilitate its public image or gain favor with government regulators. "There have been an estimated 100 million deaths due to tobacco over the last century. How can we trust the companies that caused this human disaster" said World Health Organization (WHO) tobacco-control expert Armando Peruga. "By appearing to offer a solution with one hand, while continuing to create mass destruction with the other, the tobacco industry is trying to regain the respectability it lost long ago. The manufacturers of cigarettes and other tobacco products cannot be legitimate partners in any public health discussion" (Fleck 2014).

Federal Regulation of Vaping Products

The big tobacco companies' growing involvement in the vaping industry also caught the attention of the U.S. Food and Drug Administration (FDA). Beginning in the 1960s, federal lawmakers and agencies enacted regulations aimed at curbing the abuses of the tobacco industry and informing consumers about the dangers of smoking. They banned cigarette advertising and promotional messages that targeted children, required health warning labels to appear on packaging, restricted the use of flavoring in tobacco products, and prohibited smoking in public places. Combined with antismoking advocacy and educational campaigns, these measures led to a steady decline in cigarette smoking in the United States.

E-cigarettes were not subject to the same regulations as combustible cigarettes. Vaping proponents presented e-cigarettes as a safer alternative to cigarettes that could help smokers quit. They called on federal authorities to support e-cigarette innovation and promote vaping as a tobacco harm reduction strategy and smoking-cessation tool. They argued that switching cigarette smokers to e-cigarettes would destroy the tobacco industry and benefit public health. In the absence of regulation, however, some e-cigarette manufacturers adopted deceptive tactics that had once been used by the tobacco industry, such as minimizing health risks, misleading consumers about nicotine content, and introducing sweet flavors and colorful social-media campaigns designed to appeal to young people.

These tactics contributed to a surge in youth vaping. One survey found that the percentage of high-school seniors who vaped nicotine during the previous 30 days nearly doubled from 11 percent in 2017 to 21 percent in 2018—the largest one-year increase in adolescent substance use ever recorded (Hiltzik 2018). Across the United States, teachers and administrators reported students "Juuling" in school bathrooms between classes. On social media, teenagers posted videos of vaping tricks or tips for hiding e-cigarette use from adults. The popularity of vaping made tobacco use seem trendy, rebellious, and cool again. "In just a few years, vaping has wiped out two decades of work getting teens to quit (or never start) cigarette smoking," said *Mother Jones* writer Kevin Drum (Hiltzik 2018).

Public health officials expressed alarm at the increase in youth vaping, claiming that the trend threatened to cause a new generation of Americans to become addicted to nicotine. Although experts generally acknowledged that vaping involved fewer health risks than cigarette smoking, they insisted that it was far from harmless. "Nicotine exposure during adolescence can harm the developing brain—which continues to develop until about age 25," said U.S. Surgeon General Jerome Adams. "Nicotine exposure during adolescence can impact learning, memory, and attention. Using nicotine in adolescence can also increase risk for future addiction to other drugs" (Hiltzik 2018). In addition, some studies suggested that young people who experimented with vaping were more likely to begin smoking cigarettes than teens who never tried e-cigarettes.

Describing youth vaping as an "epidemic," FDA Commissioner Scott Gottlieb responded by increasing enforcement of minimum-age rules prohibiting the sale of nicotine products to minors. He also ordered manufacturers of the top five e-cigarette brands to submit detailed plans for preventing underage use of their products. If these measures proved ineffective, Gottlieb warned that the FDA would consider pulling vaping products from the market or banning the sale of flavored e-liquids. Antismoking advocates urged the FDA to place the same restrictions on e-cigarettes as other tobacco products, including advertising bans, warning labels, and prohibitions on vaping in public places. Vaping supporters criticized the proposed regulations, arguing that they would restrict the availability of e-cigarettes as a reduced-harm alternative or smoking-cessation tool for adult cigarette smokers.

Critics claimed that tougher regulation of vaping products would benefit the big tobacco companies by forcing people to continue smoking. "If a crackdown reduces the number of smokers switching to e-cigs, it would likely be bad for public health but financially a benefit for public tobacco companies," said industry analyst Michael Lavery (Aiello 2018). Vaping proponents also noted that compliance with stricter regulations was likely to be complex, time consuming, and expensive. They argued that big tobacco companies had the resources and experience to deal with such regulations, while small, independent e-cigarette manufacturers would likely be forced out of the market. In the absence of dynamic, innovative competition, analysts predicted that the tobacco companies would deemphasize e-cigarettes in favor of more profitable products. "The cigarette companies make all their money in cigarettes—that's the high-margin business where they have scale," Lavery explained. "They all have smaller vape or e-cigarette businesses, but they are still in investment mode. They make little or no money there and, in some cases, lose money" (Aiello 2018).

Even though the tobacco industry potentially stood to benefit from an FDA crackdown on vaping, public health officials argued that protecting consumers from harm took precedence over protecting independent e-cigarette producers. "The tobacco industry is already overpowering the smaller e-cigarette manufacturers as a result of market competition and in the absence of significant regulation," Peruga stated. "E-cigarette regulations are designed to protect public health and to be effective. They should be applied to all market players, large or small, the same way other products are regulated" (Fleck 2014).

Further Reading

Abate, Carolyn. 2017. "Tobacco Companies Taking Over the E-Cigarette Industry." Huffington Post, February 27, 2017. https://www.huffingtonpost.com/entry/tobacco-companies-taking-over-the-e-cigarette-industry_us_58b48e02e4b0658fc20f98d0.

Aiello, Chloe. 2018. "Big Tobacco Stands to Benefit from an FDA Crackdown on E-Cigs, Analyst Says." CNBC, September 13, 2018. https://www.cnbc.com/2018/09/13/analyst-big-tobacco-stands-to-benefit-from-an-fda-crackdown-on-e-cigs.html.

Becker, Rachel. 2018. "What a Ban on E-Cigarette Flavors Could Mean for Big Tobacco." The Verge, November 9, 2018. https://www.theverge.com/2018/11/9/18080308/electronic-cigarettes-fda-flavor-ban-vaping-juul-blu-vuse-big-tobacco.

Fleck, Fiona. 2014. "Countries Vindicate Cautious Stance on E-Cigarettes." *Bulletin of the World Health Organization* 92 (12): 856, December 2014. https://www.who.int/bulletin/volumes/92/12/14-031214/en/.

Gurdus, Lizzy. 2018. "Cramer: Vaping Is Decimating the Cigarette Industry—and It Could Get Worse." CNBC, April 23, 2018. https://www.cnbc.com/2018/04/23/cramer-vaping-is-killing-the-cigarette-industry-and-it-may-get-worse.html.

Hiltzik, Michael. 2018. "A Tobacco Company Makes Juul's Founders Billionaires while Questions Rise about Their Product's Safety." *Los Angeles Times,*

December 28, 2018. https://www.latimes.com/business/hiltzik/la-fi
-hiltzik-juul-20181228-story.html.

Jain, Tanusree. 2018. "Big Tobacco Has Become Big Vape, but It's Up to the Same
Old Tricks." *Maclean's*, January 30, 2018. https://www.macleans.ca/soci-
ety/health/big-tobacco-has-become-big-vape-but-its-up-to-the-same
-old-tricks/.

LaVito, Angelica. 2018. "Altria Shutters Its E-Cigarette Brands as It Eyes Juul,
Awaits iQOS Decision." CNBC, December 7, 2018. https://www.cnbc
.com/2018/12/07/altria-closes-e-cigarette-brands-as-it-eyes-juul-awaits
-iqos-decision.html.

Mead, Theo. 2019. "How Vaping Is Disrupting the Tobacco Industry." Daily
Caller, January 23, 2019. https://dailycaller.com/2019/01/23/how-vaping
-is-disrupting-the-tobacco-industry/.

Thomas, Naomi. 2018. "U.S. Cigarette Smoking Rate Reaches New Low." CNN,
November 8, 2018. https://www.cnn.com/2018/11/08/health/cigarette
-tobacco-use-study/index.html.

Waldrep, Jordan. 2018. "Why the Maker of Marlboro Cigarettes Just Quit Part of
the Vape Market." *Forbes*, November 6, 2018. https://www.forbes.com
/sites/jordanwaldrep/2018/11/06/why-the-maker-of-marlboro-cigarettes
-just-quit-part-of-the-vape-market/#656b0c3d4d8b.

Vaping and Tobacco in American Politics

The polarized national debate over vaping often features a partisan political component. The basic philosophies of government underpinning the two major U.S. political parties largely shape their policy goals for tobacco control and regulation of e-cigarettes. In general, the Republican Party presents itself as pro-business and supports the vaping industry as a source of innovation and economic growth. Republicans also prefer to minimize government interference in citizens' lives, which means that they generally favor low taxes and limited regulation. The Democratic Party, on the other hand, tends to promote a more active role for government in advancing the interests of the American people and helping those in need. Most Democrats want to regulate e-cigarettes to prevent youth vaping and protect consumers from potential health risks.

Tobacco Money and Political Influence

The positions of the two political parties on e-cigarettes reflect their longstanding positions on tobacco control. In most cases, Democrats led the federal government's efforts to curb the abuses of the tobacco industry and protect consumers from the health hazards of cigarette smoking. In

1994, for instance, Democratic representative Henry Waxman of California invited top executives from the seven largest tobacco companies to testify before Congress, where they falsely claimed that nicotine was not addictive. In 2009, Democrats were the primary sponsors of the Family Smoking Prevention and Tobacco Control Act, which gave the U.S. Food and Drug Administration (FDA) authority to regulate tobacco products. Although the legislation received some bipartisan support, most of the opposition came from Republican members of Congress from tobacco-farming states, such as Georgia, Kentucky, North Carolina, and Virginia.

Historically, the Republican Party's pro-business, anti-regulation ideology has tended to attract more financial support from large corporations—including the big tobacco companies—in the form of campaign contributions. From 1990 through 2016, 74 percent of all tobacco industry political donations went to Republicans, for a total of $57 million (Glenza 2017). "We supported the Republican party not only because of its pro-business platform, but because the party wants to take the country in a direction most Americans want to go," said Joseph S. Helewicz, a spokesperson for the Brown and Williamson tobacco company. "That includes less government, less red tape, a balanced budget, and other key planks in the Republican platform" (Fritsch 1995). During the 2014 and 2016 elections, the percentage of tobacco industry contributions that went to Republican candidates increased to 84 percent (Glenza 2017).

Critics assert that the tobacco companies use political contributions to buy influence with legislators and convince them to pursue policies that benefit the industry. "Tobacco industry influence in Washington is pervasive, in many different ways," said Senator Richard Blumenthal, a Democrat from Connecticut who participated in the state lawsuits against the tobacco industry in the 1990s. "They have an active presence on the Hill, they meet frequently with administrative agencies, on hugely significant issues such as regulation of e-cigarettes, tobacco packaging, and warnings" (Glenza 2017).

Tobacco industry expenditures on political activities increased significantly following the 2016 election of Republican President Donald Trump. The two leading U.S. tobacco companies, Altria and Reynolds American, ranked among the largest donors to Trump's inauguration, giving a combined total of $1.5 million (Schouten and O'Donnell 2017). Each of the tobacco giants hired more than a dozen lobbying firms to represent their interests with federal legislators and regulators, and together with other cigarette makers and industry groups spent $4.7 million on lobbying during the first quarter of 2017 (Myers 2017). "We will continue our efforts to educate elected officials on matters that are important to our consumers, our shareholders, and other stakeholders," declared Reynolds American spokesperson David Howard. "It is particularly important to do so with people new in government roles who may not have the background and information about the issues" (Schouten and O'Donnell 2017).

Upon taking office, Trump filled several high-profile offices—including the secretary of Health and Human Services, the attorney general, and the surgeon general—with individuals who had close ties to the tobacco industry. As part of a proposed health care reform bill, Republicans in Congress attempted to cut funding for antismoking education programs offered through the U.S. Centers for Disease Control and Prevention (CDC) and to eliminate smoking-cessation coverage for low-income Americans through the federal Medicaid insurance program. Critics contended that such measures threatened to reverse decades of progress in reducing U.S. cigarette-smoking rates. "With the new Trump administration and Congress trying to roll back health and safety regulations, generally the tobacco industry is seizing the opportunity to mount its own assault on the programs and policies that have reduced smoking in this country," said Vince Wilmore of the Campaign for Tobacco-Free Kids (Glenza 2017).

The Fight over Vaping Regulation

In May 2016, the FDA finalized its deeming rules, which gave the agency authority to regulate e-cigarettes as tobacco products. The new regulations required manufacturers of vaping products to provide lists of ingredients, place nicotine warning labels on packaging and advertising materials, and stop offering free samples at promotional events. It also established a federal minimum age of 18 for the purchase of vaping products. The most controversial provision required e-cigarette manufacturers to submit premarket review applications for all components and parts and obtain FDA approval to remain on the market. Supporters argued that the review process would allow the FDA to assess the health risks associated with e-cigarettes, ensure product safety, and protect consumers. Yet the rules included an exemption for tobacco products that had existed in equivalent form prior to 2007, which applied to most combustible cigarettes.

Pro-vaping advocates argued that subjecting e-cigarettes to the complex, expensive, and time-consuming premarket approval process would destroy the vaping industry and force small, independent manufacturers out of business. They claimed that the requirement would deny smokers access to a potentially lifesaving reduced-harm alternative while exempting tobacco products proven to be far more harmful. "Reasonable product standards that actually help make the products better, help instill consumer confidence, that would be fine," said Greg Conley, president of the American Vaping Association. "But what the FDA has proposed is not regulation; it is prohibition for 99 percent of products on the market today" (Selig, Bender, and Cannaviccio 2018). Some critics charged that government officials protected the tobacco industry from competition to maintain the flow of campaign contributions, lobbying expenditures, and revenue from cigarette taxes.

In response to concerns expressed by vaping supporters, Representatives Tom Cole (R-OK) and Sanford Bishop (D-GA) introduced HR 1136, known as the Cole-Bishop Amendment. The bill proposed to change the effective date of the premarket review requirement to allow all existing e-cigarettes to remain on the market. In effect, it would extend the grandfather exemption to include vaping products as well as traditional tobacco products. The Cole-Bishop Amendment received vocal support from vaping enthusiasts and e-cigarette makers, who argued that it would promote competition and save lives. It also received vocal opposition from public health organizations, who claimed it would hamper the FDA's ability to prevent youth vaping and protect public health. In the end, Democrats in Congress managed to kill the bill.

In 2017, Trump appointed Scott Gottlieb as the new FDA commissioner. Vaping supporters praised the choice, noting that Gottlieb had previously worked for the pro-vaping American Enterprise Institute and served on the board of directors for the Kure vape shop franchise. In July 2017, Gottlieb gave the vaping industry a reprieve from the deeming regulations by postponing the premarket application deadline for e-cigarettes from 2018 to 2022. Although Gottlieb continued to express support for e-cigarettes as a reduced-harm alternative for adult smokers, he grew increasingly concerned about what he described as an "epidemic" of youth vaping. By late 2018, he ordered the leading e-cigarette manufacturers to devise plans to prevent underage use of their products and threatened to pull products off the market if they refused to comply. Gottlieb also considered banning the sale of flavored e-liquids, which he viewed as a major factor increasing the appeal of vaping for teenagers.

As the Republican-led FDA cracked down on the vaping industry, the Trump administration proposed extending tobacco "user fees" to e-cigarettes. The fees essentially amounted to a federal tax on vaping products, which would make them more expensive for consumers. Administration officials claimed that the fees would discourage teen vaping as well as generate $100 million annually to fund the FDA's regulatory programs and educational campaigns to combat underage tobacco use. Vaping supporters criticized the proposed tax, asserting that raising the cost of e-cigarettes would cause more people to smoke cigarettes and thus be detrimental to public health. "If the intent here is to achieve tax parity between cigarettes and vapor products, that is a huge mistake and a massive giveaway to Big Tobacco," said Liz Mair of the nonprofit group Vapers United. "If your concern is improving public health, . . . your policy should generally be to keep vapor taxes much lower than cigarette taxes to incentivize people to try to quit smoking using them" (Boehm 2019).

Some vaping advocates argued that the government should increase cigarette taxes to create incentives for people to switch to e-cigarettes. In addition to serving as a harm-reduction measure and reducing health care costs from smoking-related diseases, higher cigarette taxes could also reduce the gateway effect of teenage vapers eventually starting to smoke. Pro-vaping supporters also objected to bans on vaping in public places and restrictions on sales of flavored e-liquids enacted by many city and state governments. "When it comes to other legal drugs, we don't require that products intended for adults be made unpalatable to minors, even if they're not supposed to be getting their hands on them," wrote *Slate* contributor Jacob Grier. "Teen drinking is a serious problem—the Centers for Disease Control and Prevention estimates that excessive drinking causes more than 4,300 deaths among the underaged each year, which is approximately 4,300 more deaths than can be attributed to teen vaping—but we don't address this by banning adult beverages that young people also find appealing" (Grier 2019).

Grier asserted that the FDA's repeated warnings about youth vaping created "an alarmist political climate that has put e-cigarettes under attack" (Grier 2019), leading to a plethora of anti-vaping laws at all levels of government. The politicization of the vaping debate also caused widespread confusion and misunderstanding about the relative health risks of e-cigarettes. A survey of public attitudes about vaping found that the percentage of people who viewed e-cigarettes as less harmful than combustible cigarettes decreased by 10 points from 2012 to 2017, from 45 percent to 35 percent. Meanwhile, the percentage of people who viewed e-cigarettes as equally harmful as regular cigarettes increased by the same margin. The researchers concluded that their findings "underscore the urgent need to accurately communicate the risks of e-cigarettes to the public" (Bracho-Sanchez 2019).

Some pro-vaping activists sought to mobilize the estimated 10 million vapers in the United States as a political force to advocate for vaping rights. Many outspoken vaping enthusiasts were former cigarette smokers who credited e-cigarettes with enabling them to quit. "People who had literally been smoking for decades, all of a sudden are never having another cigarette again," said Cheryl Richter, a vape shop owner and co-founder of the National Vapers Club. "We've been kind of bullied outside for a very long time. We're told we smell, and we're going to die. And get away from my kids with that [cigarette]. So now we're vaping and we're very proud of ourselves. *Extremely* proud of ourselves" (Sottile 2014).

The Consumer Advocates for Smoke-Free Alternatives Association, the American Vaping Association, NOT Blowing Smoke, and various state pro-vaping organizations worked to educate people about the benefits of vaping over smoking, encourage lawmakers to oppose vaping taxes and regulations, raise money to fund scientific research, and organize voters in support of vaping rights. Political activist Grover Norquist, founder of Americans for Tax Reform, predicted that e-cigarette users would become a potent political force. "Vaping is not a product. It's a movement," he stated. "It is a community, it is a political movement in support of a community, and it's changing the country in very good ways" (Barro 2018).

Further Reading

Barro, Josh. 2018. "The Best Way to Capture Public-Health Benefits from Vaping? Make Cigarettes Harder to Get." *New York Magazine*, December 20, 2018. http://nymag.com/intelligencer/2018/12/to-reduce-ill-effects-of -vaping-restrict-cigarettes.html.

Boehm, Eric. 2019. "Trump Wants to Tax Your Juul." *Reason*, March 12, 2019. https://reason.com/blog/2019/03/12/trump-wants-to-tax-your-juul.

Bracho-Sanchez, Edith. 2019. "More Americans Think E-Cigarettes Are Harmful, Study Says." CNN, March 29, 2019. https://www.cnn.com/2019/03/29 /health/ecigarette-cigarette-risks-study/index.html.

Fritsch, Jane. 1995. "Tobacco Companies Pump Cash into Republican Party's Coffers." *New York Times*, September 13, 1995. https://www.nytimes.com /1995/09/13/us/tobacco-companies-pump-cash-into-republican-party-s -coffers.html.

Glenza, Jessica. 2017. "Tobacco Companies Tighten Hold on Washington under Trump." *Guardian*, July 13, 2017. https://www.theguardian.com/world /2017/jul/13/tobacco-industry-trump-administration-ties.

Grier, Jacob. 2019. "We Are Completely Overreacting to Vaping." *Slate*, January 29, 2019. https://slate.com/technology/2019/01/vaping-is-good-anti-smoker -bias.html.

Mitchell, Dan. 2018. "The Political Economy of Vaping." Truth on the Market, October 19, 2018. https://truthonthemarket.com/2018/10/19/the-politi cal-economy-of-vaping/.

Myers, Matthew L. 2017. "Tobacco Companies Gave $1.5 Million to Trump Inaugural and Ramped Up Lobbying." Campaign for Tobacco-Free Kids, April 21, 2017. https://www.tobaccofreekids.org/press-releases/2017_04 _21_trump.

Schouten, Fredreka, and Jayne O'Donnell. 2017. "E-Cigarette Industry Gains Allies in Regulation Fight." *USA Today*, April 26, 2017. https://www.usa today.com/story/news/politics/2017/04/26/e-cigarette-industry -gains-allies-regulation-fight/100939604/.

Selig, Roni, Maddie Bender, and Davide Cannaviccio. 2018. "Juul and the Vape Debate: Choosing between Smokers and Teens." CNN, August 9, 2018. https://www.cnn.com/2018/08/09/health/juul-teen-vape-debate/index .html.

Sottile, Leah. 2014. "The Right to Vape." *Atlantic*, October 8, 2014. https://www .theatlantic.com/health/archive/2014/10/the-right-to-vape/381145/.

CHAPTER FOUR

Profiles

This section provides illuminating biographical profiles of important figures in the vaping controversy and the larger tobacco-control movement, including Juul creators Adam Bowen and James Monsees, pro-vaping activists Aaron Biebert and Bill Godshall, tobacco-control advocates Stanton Glantz and Henry Waxman, and federal regulators David Kessler and Scott Gottlieb.

Aaron Biebert (1982–)

Pro-vaping activist and filmmaker

Aaron Biebert was born in Milwaukee, Wisconsin, on March 10, 1982. The oldest of eight children in his family, Biebert grew up in Inver Grove Heights, Minnesota. He attended St. Croix Lutheran High School in St. Paul, where he participated in theatrical productions. He met his future wife, Jennifer, backstage after one performance. They married in 2004 and eventually had two children, son Frederick and daughter Sydney. Biebert attended Wisconsin Lutheran College in Milwaukee, where he played football and earned a degree in business administration with a minor in art.

After college, Biebert launched several entrepreneurial business ventures, including a mortgage brokerage firm and a medical services company. In 2010, he established Attention Era Media, a commercial production company. Biebert originally produced music videos, sports highlight films, marketing materials, and social media storytelling movies. After one of Biebert's friends died of lung cancer, Biebert began conducting research into nicotine addiction, smoking cessation, and the resources available to help people give up cigarettes. Upon reading a World Health Organization (WHO) report predicting that a billion people would die prematurely during the twenty-first century due to the harmful effects of cigarette smoking, Biebert concluded that smoking is "probably one of the biggest health crises in the history of the world" (Malmin 2018).

Biebert also learned more about vaping, which many critics portrayed as equally dangerous as cigarette smoking. Through interviews with medical experts and vapers around the world, he became convinced that vaping was a healthier alternative that could help smokers quit or at least reduce their chances of developing smoking-related illnesses. Biebert encountered many former smokers who believed that the tobacco industry and its allies in the government and media were actively trying to prevent the public from learning about the potential health benefits of vaping. "I initially thought that vaping looked like some hipster way to keep smoking indoors," he acknowledged. "Years later, some friends educated me more on the topic. They sounded like conspiracy theorists with talk about how big business and government interests were interfering with this cheap, drug-free alternative that is helping many people quit smoking" ("Q&A" 2018).

Biebert decided to explore the controversy surrounding vaping in a documentary film called *A Billion Lives* (2016). The project set out to expose what Biebert viewed as a corrupt scheme perpetrated by the tobacco industry, pharmaceutical companies, government agencies, medical professionals, and anti-cancer charities to suppress vaping as a potentially lifesaving alternative to cigarette smoking. "If smoking disappeared tomorrow, there would be nearly a trillion dollars of lost revenue," he asserted. "Giant companies would fail. Massive charity organizations would lose their donations. Government programs would shut down. That's why vaping has been attacked. There's no other explanation. The science is clear. Our movie shows that the propaganda being disseminated by the government is very misleading" ("Q&A" 2018).

According to Biebert, the pharmaceutical industry is largely responsible for the anti-vaping campaign. "They earn billions of dollars by producing nicotine gum, patches, and sprays, along with other smoking cessation drugs such as Chantix and Wellbutrin. These profits are at risk as vaping increases in popularity as an alternative to smoking," he explained. "There are billions of dollars at stake with sales of their cancer drugs, chemotherapy, and prescription medications. Simply put, smoking is a lifeline for Big Pharma's profits" (Meyer 2016). Biebert also claimed that the media promoted anti-vaping messages because they depended on advertising revenues from pharmaceutical companies, which ranked as the second-leading source of ad spending in the United States.

A Billion Lives analyzed studies suggesting that vaping was more dangerous than smoking. Biebert disputed the results, claiming that the tests heated vaping liquids to such high temperatures that human beings would be unable to ingest them. "That'd be like saying bread causes more cancer than cigarettes if you toast the thing to black every time," he stated. "No human would eat burnt crust all day every day, but you could make a case that bread causes more cancer than cigarettes" (Mueller 2016).

Nevertheless, such studies convinced the U.S. Food and Drug Administration (FDA) to propose strict regulations on the vaping industry. In December 2015, Biebert gave a speech before President Barack Obama and the White House Office of Management and Budget (OMB) opposing the regulations. "The best estimate is that e-cigarettes are around 95 percent less harmful than smoking; nearly half the population don't realize e-cigarettes are much less harmful than smoking; and there's no evidence so far that e-cigarettes are acting as a route into smoking for children or non-smokers," he contended (Biebert 2015).

Although Biebert does not smoke or vape, he has emerged as a leading activist in the movement to promote vaping as a safer alternative that holds the potential to save the lives of many cigarette smokers. "At the end of the day, this isn't really a political issue; it's just should people live or die, should they have the truth or not," he stated. "And I think we can all agree they should have the truth, and they should be allowed to live if they want" (Mueller 2016).

Further Reading

Biebert, Aaron. 2015. "Speech to the White House Office of Management and Budget." *A Billion Lives,* December 11, 2015. https://www.facebook.com/notes/a-billion-lives/speech-to-white-house-omb/1015436971836356.

Malmin, Bard. 2018. "A Billion Lives and the Winston Man: The Exclusive Interview." *Vapetrotter News,* March 8, 2018. https://www.vapetrotter.com/news/a-billion-lives-the-winston-man-the-exclusive-interview/.

Meyer, Jared. 2016. "Government Puts Tobacco Interests above a Billion Lives." *Forbes,* October 2, 2016. https://www.forbes.com/sites/jaredmeyer/2016/10/02/government-puts-tobacco-interests-above-a-billion-lives/#57d588256424.

Mueller, Matt. 2016. "A Billion Lives Global Vaping Doc Makes U.S. Premier in Milwaukee." *On Milwaukee,* August 5, 2016. https://onmilwaukee.com/movies/articles/abillionlives.html.

"Q&A with Director Aaron Biebert." 2018. *A Billion Lives.* https://abillionlives.com/qa-with-director-aaron-biebert/.

Vape Organics. 2015. "Inspiration Series, Part IV: Aaron Biebert." December 8, 2015. http://pureorganicvapors.com/general/aaron-biebert-interview/.

Adam Bowen (1976?–) and James Monsees (1980?–)

Inventors of the Juul e-cigarette

Adam Bowen was born around 1976 in Tucson, Arizona. After receiving a bachelor's degree in physics from Pomona College in Claremont, California, in 1998, he went on to earn a master's degree in mechanical engineering and product design from Stanford University in 2005. James Monsees was born around 1980 in St. Louis, Missouri. He earned a bachelor's degree in physics and studio art from Kenyon College in Gambier, Ohio, in 2002, followed by a master's degree in product design from Stanford University in 2006.

Bowen and Monsees met as graduate students at Stanford in 2003. One day, while they were taking a smoke break outside the product design lab, they began discussing the shortcomings of cigarettes. "We're relatively smart people and we're standing out here burning sticks," Monsees recalled. "We kind of love this ritual and these products in certain ways. But we had a lot of problems with it. What would happen if we try to design a better experience for ourselves?" (Montoya 2015). This idea formed the basis of a design project for their master's thesis.

Bowen and Monsees interviewed fellow students on campus to gain insights into their smoking habits and the elements of cigarettes that they liked and disliked. They also took advantage of the vast collection of tobacco industry documents made available online as part of the Master Settlement Agreement, which required the tobacco companies to pay billions of dollars to reimburse the states for the costs of treating smoking-related illnesses. The graduate students reviewed patent applications, market analyses, scientific research findings, and minutes of board meetings. "We did a ton of research on why the industry had evolved to where it was at that time," Monsees recalled. "We became fascinated with how big the industry was and how small the innovation rate seemed to be relative to that market size. It seemed like a standout opportunity in product design to work on something that would have an impact" ("James Monsees" 2014). The partners built and tested hundreds of prototypes in their search for a breakthrough improvement in cigarette design.

Around this time, Chinese inventor Hon Lik patented the first modern electronic cigarette, which worked by heating a liquid containing nicotine to create an inhalable vapor. After earning their master's degrees, Bowen and Monsees formed a startup company, Ploom, in San Francisco to continue developing smokeless cigarette products. One of their early designs, the Pax vaporizer, heated loose-leaf tobacco or cannabis to form a vapor. In 2011, they sold Ploom and launched a new company, Pax Labs. As the U.S. market for e-cigarettes grew, the partners turned their attention toward streamlining the design of early vaping devices, which tended to be large and unattractive, and improving their function. "The products that were on the market before then were sort of wooden boxes, weird stuff," Monsees noted (Montoya 2015). "Our belief is this: If you really want to satisfy smokers, if you really want to make an alternative and make cigarettes obsolete, you need to provide something that is an overall better experience—something that is better in every way" (Yakowicz 2018).

In 2015, Bowen and Monsees introduced a revolutionary new e-cigarette called the Juul. The simple, sleek, elegant design resembled a USB memory stick, with one part containing a heating element and a rechargeable battery, and a separate cartridge or "pod" containing e-liquid. Juul pods came in eight flavors—including mango, cucumber, fruit, crème, and mint— and each pod contained about as much nicotine as a pack of cigarettes. With the help of a colorful marketing campaign centered on social media, sales of the Juul e-cigarette took off. In 2017, the creators left Pax Labs and spun off Juul Labs as an independent company, with Bowen as chief technology officer and Monsees as chief product officer. During 2018, as sales more than tripled to reach an estimated $2 billion, the company grew from 225 employees to 1,500 (Sherman 2019). By the fall of 2018, Juul accounted for 75 percent of e-cigarette sales in the United States.

Juul's astronomical growth raised concerns among antismoking groups and federal regulators, who attributed it largely to the device's popularity among teenagers. Bowen and Monsees insisted that they never intended for Juul to initiate underage youth to vaping and expose them to nicotine. "It is an issue we desperately want to resolve," Monsees said. "It doesn't do us any favors. Any underage consumers using this product are absolutely a negative for our business. We don't want them. We will never market to them. We never have" (Chaykowski 2018). With the U.S. Food and Drug Administration (FDA) launching an investigation into Juul and threatening to impose regulations, Bowen and Monsees took action to prevent youth access, including changing their marketing approach to emphasize adult former smokers, removing popular sweet flavors from retail stores, strengthening age verification for online sales, and launching a $30 million educational campaign.

In December 2018, Bowen and Monsees sold a 35 percent stake in Juul Labs to Altria, the tobacco company that produces the industry-leading Marlboro cigarette brand, for $12.8 billion. Juul stood to benefit from

Altria's marketing reach and political connections, while Altria gained a presence in the e-cigarette industry. Although the deal made Bowen and Monsees billionaires, critics argued that it also detracted from Juul's credibility as an antismoking company.

Further Reading

Chaykowski, Kathleen. 2018. "The Disturbing Focus of Juul's Early Marketing Campaigns." *Forbes,* November 16, 2018. https://www.forbes.com/sites/kathleenchaykowski/2018/11/16/the-disturbing-focus-of-juuls-early-marketing-campaigns/#59c924f614f9.

"James Monsees: Co-Founder and CEO of Ploom." 2014. IdeaMensch, April 11, 2014. https://ideamensch.com/james-monsees/.

Lee, Seung. 2018. "Juul Labs Co-Founders Say They're Working toward a World without Smokers." *San Jose Mercury News,* September 12, 2018. https://www.mercurynews.com/2018/09/12/juul-labs-co-founders-say-theyre-working-toward-a-world-without-smokers/.

Montoya, Gabriel. 2015. "Pax Labs: Origins with James Monsees." Social Underground, January 2015. https://socialunderground.com/2015/01/pax-ploom-origins-future-james-monsees/.

Sherman, Natalie. 2019. "Juul: The Rise of a $38 Billion E-Cigarette Phenomenon." BBC News, January 6, 2019. https://www.bbc.com/news/business-46654063.

Yakowicz, Will. 2018. "Inside Juul: The Most Promising, and Controversial, Vape Company in America." *Inc.,* September 24, 2018. https://www.inc.com/will-yakowicz/2018-private-titans-juul-labs-vaporizer-nicotine-electronic-cigarettes.html.

Stefan Didak (1970?–)

Pro-vaping activist and founder of NOT Blowing Smoke

Stefan Didak was born around 1970 in the Netherlands, where he spent most of his youth. By his late teens, he became interested in the emerging fields of software development, computer-generated imagery, 3D animation, digital post-production, and virtual reality. Didak launched his first entrepreneurial venture, Animagic, in 1989. He went on to establish several other companies that used sophisticated computer technology to help clients turn ideas into commercial products. In 2000, he founded mantiCORE Labs with the goal of "building bridges between human creativity and technology" ("About" 2019). Didak also began dividing his time between Europe and northern California around this time. In 2012, he founded businesses called Ignyter and Ignytion. During his career in computer graphics, Didak became known for his "world famous home office setup," which featured large banks of high-tech computer monitors. "In the midst of the flashing LED's and lights of a collection of workstations, network switches, disk arrays, and gadgets I feel right at home," he stated ("About" 2019).

A longtime cigarette smoker, Didak switched to vaping in 2012 and noticed many positive impacts on his health. Over the next few years, he emerged as a vocal advocate of e-cigarettes as a reduced-harm alternative to combustible cigarettes and an effective smoking-cessation tool. He claimed that vaping had the potential to save the lives of millions of smokers as well as people exposed to secondhand smoke. Didak contended that public health officials misled consumers about the health effects of e-cigarettes to protect the interests of the tobacco lobby, and he fought to keep vapor products available and accessible to adult users.

In 2014, the U.S. Food and Drug Administration (FDA) proposed new "deeming" regulations that extended the agency's authority over tobacco products to include e-cigarettes. Under the proposed rules, e-cigarette manufacturers would be required to submit a premarket tobacco application demonstrating the safety and public health benefits of their products to receive FDA approval to sell them in the United States. Didak and other pro-vaping advocates argued that the difficulty and expense of the premarket approval process would cripple the vaping industry and cause independent e-cigarette producers to go out of business. The reduced availability of e-cigarettes, in turn, would force consumers to obtain nicotine from combustible cigarettes, to the detriment of public health. Didak also pointed out that the FDA regulations included an exemption for tobacco products that were introduced before February 2007, which applied only to combustible cigarettes. He asserted that the proposed deeming rules put the interests of tobacco companies above those of consumers by stifling innovation and suppressing the development of reduced-harm alternatives.

In 2015, Didak founded a pro-vaping advocacy organization called NOT Blowing Smoke to oppose the FDA regulations. According to its website, its purpose was "to ensure continued and affordable access to vapor products in order to help smokers and those around them lead improved lives, free from the death and disease caused by combustible cigarettes. Our focus is on raising public awareness through educational and promotional campaigns as well as actions to represent the interests of both industry stakeholders and consumers" (NOT Blowing Smoke 2018). Didak opposed restrictions on vaping in blog entries, social media posts, articles, interviews, and testimony at public hearings. The NOT Blowing

Smoke website featured news and information about the FDA's proposed deeming regulations as well as a guide for voters and a calendar of meetings, protests, and opportunities for vaping supporters to take action. Didak and NOT Blowing Smoke came under criticism from antismoking advocates, who claimed that the pro-vaping forces cited research funded by the tobacco industry to support their position and attacked independent findings suggesting e-cigarettes may not be safe.

In 2017, Didak and other vaping advocates celebrated when FDA Commissioner Scott Gottlieb gave e-cigarette manufacturers a reprieve by extending the premarket application deadline to 2022. Yet the delay of the federal regulations, combined with an increase in vaping among teenagers, convinced many state and local governments to enact their own laws restricting vapor products. Many of the proposed laws targeted flavored e-liquids, which public health organizations blamed for attracting young people to e-cigarettes. Didak actively opposed flavor bans, arguing that many former smokers relied upon flavored e-liquids to help them kick the cigarette habit. "Without the availability of flavors, the chances of people relapsing back to smoking or just smoking because of convenience becomes greater," he explained, "which is why prohibition on availability and accessibility of flavored vapor products is contrary to good harm reduction strategies" (Castle 2018).

Didak also rejected the idea that sweet flavors appealed only to children. "Adults like flavors as much as kids do," he declared, "and while the argument of 'no adult would vape bubblegum' may resonate with non-vapers and non-smokers alike, the truth is that many of us have and still do" (Castle 2018). He pointed out that many other adult-oriented products—such as coffee and vodka—come in sweet flavors without critics complaining that they might appeal to kids. Despite Didak's efforts, San Francisco passed an ordinance in 2017 banning the sale of flavored tobacco products. Didak and other pro-vaping activists responded by forming an organization called Let's Be Real and collecting enough voter signatures to force the city to hold a referendum on repealing the flavor ban. When he is not organizing on behalf of the right to vape, Didak enjoys photography, travel, restaurants, cats, and Corvettes. He and his wife, Sallie Goetsch, reside primarily in Oakley, California.

Further Reading

"About." 2019. StefanDidak.com, http://www.stefandidak.com/about/.
"Biography." 2015. FDARegs.com, http://fdaregs.info/team/stefan-didak/.

Castle, John. 2018. "Flavor Ban: Stefan Didak on San Francisco's Prop E." Vape News, June 4, 2018. https://vapenews.com/vape-news/interview-stefan -didak-on-san-franciscos-prop-e/.

Gross, Liza. 2017. "Smoke Screen: Big Vape Is Copying Big Tobacco's Playbook." The Verge, November 16, 2017. https://www.theverge.com/2017/11/16/16 658358/vape-lobby-vaping-health-risks-nicotine-big-tobacco-marketing.

NOT Blowing Smoke. 2018. http://notblowingsmoke.org/.

Stanton Glantz (1946–)

Tobacco control researcher and vocal critic of vaping

Stanton Arnold Glantz was born in Cleveland, Ohio, in 1946. His father, Louis Glantz, worked as an insurance agent, while his mother, Frieda Glantz, sold real estate. During his youth, he earned the prestigious rank of Eagle Scout in the Boy Scouts of America. In 1957, the Soviet Union's successful launch of the first artificial satellite into orbit sparked Glantz's interest in science and engineering. After earning a bachelor's degree in aerospace engineering from the University of Cincinnati in 1969, he served as a trainee with the National Aeronautics and Space Administration (NASA). Glantz continued his education at Stanford University in California, earning a master's degree in applied mechanics in 1970 followed by a PhD three years later. His early research focused on creating mathematical models to understand the mechanics of the human heart. Around the time he finished his doctorate, Glantz married his wife, Marsha, and they eventually had two children, Aaron and Freida.

In 1977, Glantz became a professor of medicine in the cardiology division at the University of California, San Francisco (UCSF). The following year, he joined the tobacco-control movement by campaigning for a California ballot initiative to create nonsmoking sections in restaurants. Although the campaign was unsuccessful, Glantz became an antismoking activist and a co-founder of Americans for Nonsmokers Rights. "I was one of the people who got the whole clean-air movement going in California," he acknowledged. "It is very gratifying to go places that are smoke-free now" (Bach 2009). Glantz also shifted the focus of his academic research to study the health effects of tobacco use. At a time when the powerful tobacco companies denied that nicotine was addictive and smoking caused lung cancer, Glantz worked to expose their deceptive marketing tactics and political spending. He eventually became director of the Center for Tobacco Control Research and Education at UCSF, overseeing the work of a team of researchers who provided evidence to support antismoking laws.

In 1982, Glantz obtained a bootleg copy of *Death in the West,* a documentary film that contrasted advertising images of the rugged Marlboro cowboy with footage of real cowboys who were dying of smoking-related illnesses. Philip Morris, the manufacturer of Marlboro cigarettes, had sued to block distribution of the film, which also featured interviews in which tobacco executives acknowledged the health risks of smoking. Glantz arranged for the movie to air at a public health seminar and on a San Francisco television station. He and other antismoking activists later turned it into an educational program to prevent adolescents from using tobacco products.

In May 1994, one month after the heads of the seven largest U.S. tobacco companies testified before Congress that nicotine was not addictive, Glantz received a mysterious delivery at his UCSF office. The two large boxes—addressed to him from "Mr. Butts," a character from the *Doonesbury* comic strip who gave cigarettes to kids—contained 4,000 pages of sensitive documents from inside the Brown and Williamson Tobacco Company, producer of the Kool, Lucky Strike, and Pall Mall cigarette brands. The documents contained incriminating evidence proving that the tobacco industry had not only known about the addictive capacity of nicotine and the health risks of smoking for decades, but had also engaged in a coordinated effort to conceal that information from consumers and government regulators. "It was stuff that everybody always sort of expected," Glantz said of the material, "but to actually see it was just mind-boggling" (Robinson 1996).

Glantz provided copies of the documents to federal officials and to a reporter for the *New York Times.* He also made them available to the public in the UCSF library. Brown and Williamson filed a lawsuit to force him to return the papers, but UCSF stood behind Glantz, and the California Supreme Court ruled in his favor. "Basically, they were trying to keep books out of the library, and universities are here to spread information, not suppress it," Glantz explained (Robinson 1996). UCSF later made the documents available on the Internet, where they formed the basis of the Truth Initiative Tobacco Industry Documents archive. It eventually grew to include 50 million pages of documents revealing the research, manufacturing, advertising, and political activities of the tobacco companies.

During the 1990s and early 2000s, Glantz became known for conducting pioneering research on the harmful effects of secondhand smoke. One influential study charted a 40 percent reduction in heart attacks in Helena, Montana, after that city passed a law in 2002 requiring all public places and work environments to be smoke-free. Known as the "Helena miracle," the study served as dramatic evidence that antismoking regulations could save lives. The results prompted the institution of smoking bans in other cities as well as on airline flights. Critics raised questions about Glantz's methods and conclusions, however, and claimed that the observed drop in heart attacks from an average of 7 to 4 per month was not statistically significant or necessarily due to a reduction in community exposure to secondhand smoke (Mason 2017). Nevertheless, Glantz continued to promote smoking bans as a way to protect the health of nonsmokers. "Your right to swing your fist ends where my nose begins," he stated. "I have never said people should be prohibited from smoking. Everybody has bad habits. But they should not be doing it in a way that poisons the air I breathe" (Bach 2009).

When electronic cigarettes began gaining popularity in the United States, Glantz emerged as a leading opponent of the new nicotine-delivery systems. He rejected claims by vaping enthusiasts that e-cigarettes offered a reduced-harm alternative to combustible cigarettes. Instead, he produced more than a dozen academic research papers that identified health risks associated with vaping. "E-cigarettes produce lower levels of cancer-causing chemicals than conventional cigarettes do," Glantz acknowledged. "But just like conventional cigarettes, they help to cause heart disease and heart attacks, lung disease, and in fact, there's growing evidence that in terms of adverse effects on the lung, e-cigarettes are actually worse than conventional cigarettes. . . . Also, because of the coils in the cigarettes, the fact that they're soldered, people get a lot of lead, cadmium, and other heavy metals" (Hobson 2018).

Glantz also disputed contentions by vaping enthusiasts that e-cigarettes helped people quit smoking. Instead, he blamed e-cigarettes for an overall rise in tobacco use among teenagers. "We've made huge progress in denormalizing tobacco use and making the cool thing to do to be a nonsmoker," Glantz stated. "Until e-cigarettes came along, total tobacco and nicotine consumption was dropping, and at least with youth it's now increasing" (Hobson 2018). Glantz's vocal stance against e-cigarettes made him a target of pro-vaping groups, who described him as a dangerous extremist who twisted facts to advance his agenda. Some of his assertions came under criticism from fellow public health experts. In a 2014 study, for instance, Glantz claimed that using e-cigarettes increased the likelihood that teenagers would smoke conventional cigarettes. Boston University tobacco-control researcher Michael Siegel, who supports vaping as a reduced-harm alternative for adult cigarette smokers, called his conclusions "fundamentally dishonest" and accused Glantz of "essentially lying to the public about the science regarding electronic cigarettes" (Siegel 2014).

Among people who share his concerns that the popularity of e-cigarettes may cause a new generation of Americans to develop nicotine addiction and harmful health effects, however, Glantz is widely respected as an antismoking crusader and consumer-protection advocate. Glantz served as an editor of the *Journal of the American College of Cardiology* for a decade. He authored or co-authored more than 200 scientific papers and nearly a dozen books, including *The Cigarette Papers* (1996) and *Tobacco War: Inside the California Battles* (2000). He has appeared in several documentary films, including *Cigarette Wars* (2011) and *Merchants of Doubt* (2014), and he is regularly interviewed on television news programs and quoted in investigative news articles about the tobacco industry and tobacco-control policies. In 2005, Glantz was elected to the prestigious Institute of Medicine. In 2017, a former postdoctoral researcher filed a complaint against Glantz for sexual harassment. Although Glantz denied the charges, UCSF paid $150,000 to settle the case out of court.

Further Reading

Bach, John. 2009. "Anti-Smoking Crusader: Stanton Glantz." *UC Magazine,* May 2009. https://magazine.uc.edu/issues/0509/crusader.html.

Hobson, Jeremy. 2018. "Vaping's Popularity—Especially among Teens—Is Cause for Concern, Researcher Says." WBUR, May 16, 2018. https://www.wbur.org/hereandnow/2018/05/16/vaping-e-cigarettes-use-teens.

Mason, Fergus. 2017. "Stanton Glantz—Expert, or Extremist?" Vaping Post, April 28, 2017. https://www.vapingpost.com/2017/04/28/stanton-glantz-expert-or-extremist/.

Robinson, Mark. 1996. "Tilting at Tobacco." *Stanford Magazine,* November/December 1996. https://stanfordmag.org/contents/tilting-at-tobacco.

Siegel, Michael. 2014. "Conclusion of New Glantz Study on Electronic Cigarettes Is Junk Science." *The Rest of the Story* (blog), March 6, 2014. http://tobaccoanalysis.blogspot.com/2014/03/conclusion-of-new-glantz-study-on.html.

Bill Godshall (1957?–)

Antismoking activist who supports vaping as tobacco harm reduction

William T. Godshall was born in Pennsylvania around 1957. He earned a bachelor's degree from Penn State University in 1980, followed by a master's degree in public health from the University of Pittsburgh in 1985. Protecting people from the dangers of cigarette smoking quickly emerged as the focus of his work in public health. In 1990, Godshall founded

Smokefree Pennsylvania, a nonprofit organization that "advocated policies to reduce tobacco smoke pollution indoors, increase cigarette taxes, reduce tobacco marketing to youth, preserve civil justice remedies for cigarette victims, expand smoking cessation services, and inform smokers that smoke-free tobacco/nicotine products are far less hazardous alternatives to cigarettes" (Electronic Cigarette Association n.d.).

Godshall's work as a tobacco-control advocate also included stints as a public health educator for the Allegheny County Health Department, director of education for the American Cancer Society in Pittsburgh, and chairman of government affairs for Stop Teenage Addiction to Tobacco. In 1999, he appeared on the famous *60 Minutes* episode that featured whistleblower Jeffrey Wigand, who informed the nation about deceptive business practices in the tobacco industry. Godshall spent the early 2000s campaigning for the passage of Pennsylvania's Clean Indoor Air Act, which banned smoking in most work environments and public places. After the law took effect in 2007, Godshall continued working to eliminate exceptions for businesses that only served people over age 18 and did not sell food, such as bars and casinos.

Among antismoking activists, Godshall became known for promoting tobacco harm reduction (THR), a public health strategy that aims to lower the risks of nicotine use by encouraging smokers to switch from combustible cigarettes to less hazardous alternatives. Although public health experts generally consider abstaining from the use of tobacco products to be the healthiest option, THR advocates argue that cutting down, switching to smokeless tobacco products, or obtaining nicotine from non-tobacco sources can offer health benefits to smokers who are unable to quit. Godshall published a series of online articles, the "Tobacco Harm Reduction Updates," to keep individual smokers, antismoking advocates, and public health officials informed about the latest developments in THR.

From the time electronic cigarettes first appeared in the United States, Godshall viewed them as a valuable THR tool. He argued that vaping had the potential to save lives by giving smokers a significantly less harmful form of nicotine delivery that replicated the experience of smoking combustible cigarettes. He pointed to research suggesting that e-cigarettes were more effective as smoking-cessation aids than the skin patches, gum, and other nicotine-replacement therapies approved by the U.S. Food and Drug Administration (FDA). Godshall also asserted that inhaling nicotine vapor did not pose health risks or create physical dependency in users. "They are saving lives," he said of e-cigarettes. "My goal has always been saving the lives of smokers" (DeJesus 2014).

After the Family Smoking Prevention and Tobacco Control Act of 2009 gave the FDA authority to regulate tobacco products, many public health organizations began pressuring agency administrators to place restrictions on e-cigarettes as well. Critics noted that e-cigarettes had not undergone rigorous scientific testing to prove their safety and efficacy, so the long-term health impacts of vaping were unknown. They also expressed concerns about the apparent popularity of vaping among teenagers, which they claimed could lead to nicotine addiction and an increased risk of using combustible cigarettes or other drugs. Godshall rejected the idea that vaping would encourage people to smoke cigarettes and instead credited e-cigarettes for reducing smoking rates among both adults and teenagers. "There are a thousand times more people who have quit smoking using vaping products than people going from [vaping products] to cigarettes," he stated (Daly 2018).

Godshall emerged as a leading opponent of the FDA's "deeming" rules, which would subject e-cigarettes to stringent federal regulations as tobacco products. He argued that the movement to restrict or ban e-cigarettes protected the financial interests of tobacco companies rather than public health. "It's simple economics," Godshall said. "E-cigarettes are to cigarettes what the automobile was to the horse and buggy industry. They weren't too happy. They wanted to ban cars" (DeJesus 2014). He also noted that vaping threatened the profits of pharmaceutical companies that produced FDA-approved nicotine-replacement therapies, which had only a 5 percent success rate in helping users quit smoking. "If you receive millions of dollars to lobby and a new product comes along that is even better at smoking cessation, what do you do?" Godshall said. "I want to keep my money flowing in from Big Pharma, so I will keep hawking their product" (DeJesus 2014).

Godshall argued against the proposed deeming regulations in testimony, articles, editorials, and blog posts. "Cigarette smokers have a human right to truthful health information and legal access to less hazardous alternatives," he wrote in official comments to the FDA. "Public health officials and agencies have an ethical duty to inform smokers that all smokefree tobacco and nicotine products are far less hazardous alternatives to cigarettes, and to keep all less hazardous alternatives legal and affordable for smokers as long as highly addictive and lethal cigarettes remain on the legal market" (Godshall 2015). Although the FDA issued deeming regulations for e-cigarettes in 2016, Godshall and other vaping advocates convinced agency officials to delay the deadline for compliance until 2022, giving e-cigarette manufacturers additional time to prove the safety and efficacy of vaping products.

In Pennsylvania, Godshall led a campaign to prevent state and local authorities from applying the Clean Indoor Air Act to vapor products. Several jurisdictions proposed bills that would ban the use of e-cigarettes in indoor public spaces where cigarette smoking was prohibited, including schools, theaters, restaurants, health care facilities, and mass transit. Supporters of the bills asserted that they protected public health, since the long-term health risks of vaping remained unclear. In response, Godshall insisted that exposure to secondhand vapor was not harmful. He also argued that elected officials should support public vaping as a smoking-cessation tool rather than sabotaging smokers' efforts to quit by forcing them to vape outdoors among cigarette smokers.

Further Reading

Daly, Jill. 2018. "Evidence on Health Effects of E-Cigarettes Is Mixed, Expert Panel Says." *Pittsburgh Post-Gazette,* January 23, 2018. https://www.post-gazette.com/news/health/2018/01/23/Evidence-on-health-effects-of-e-cigarettes-mixed-expert-committee-National-academies-Science/stories/201801230199.

DeJesus, Ivey. 2014. "E-Cigarettes: A Lone Activist Fights to Protect Them from Regulation." Penn Live, February 14, 2014. https://www.pennlive.com/midstate/index.ssf/2014/02/e-cigarettes_bill_godshall.html.

Electronic Cigarette Association. n.d. "The Facts about Electronic Cigarettes." Consumer Advocates for Smoke-free Alternatives Association. https://casaa.org/wp-content/uploads/ECA_The_Facts_About_Electronic_Cigarettes.pdf.

Godshall, William T. 2015. "Comments to the FDA Center for Tobacco Products." Consumer Advocates for Smoke-free Alternatives Association, December 2015. http://www.casaa.org/wp-content/uploads/Godshall FDAcomment-December-2015.pdf.

Sklaroff, Robert, Bill Godshall, and Stephen F. Gambescia. 2017. "Vaping Isn't Smoking, It's a Disease-Prevention Method." *The Hill,* March 17, 2017. https://thehill.com/blogs/pundits-blog/healthcare/324534-vaping-should-be-recognized-as-a-disease-prevention-public.

Scott Gottlieb (1972–)

FDA commissioner who declared youth vaping an epidemic

Scott Gottlieb was born on June 11, 1972, in East Brunswick, New Jersey, to Stanley and Marsha Gottlieb. After earning a bachelor's degree in economics from Wesleyan University in 1994, Gottlieb went on to earn a medical degree from Mt. Sinai Medical School in New York and complete his residency in internal medicine at Mt. Sinai Hospital. Rather than practicing as a physician, Gottlieb served as a health care analyst and medical consultant to investment banks and pharmaceutical companies in the late 1990s and early 2000s. He also wrote articles and served on the editorial boards of the *Journal of the American Medical Association* and the *British Medical Journal*. In 2004, Gottlieb launched a newsletter aimed at biotechnology investors called the *Forbes/Gottlieb Medical Technology Investor*. He also married Allyson Brooke Nemeroff, with whom he eventually had three daughters.

In 2005, President George W. Bush appointed Gottlieb as the deputy commissioner for medical and scientific affairs in the U.S. Food and Drug Administration (FDA), the federal agency responsible for ensuring the safety of food, dietary supplements, medications, cosmetics, and tobacco products. Critics argued that Gottlieb's financial ties to pharmaceutical companies created a conflict of interest, since his new position involved formulating government policies and regulations of pharmaceuticals. "If he's had dealings regarding companies whose products are up for review at the agency, it strikes me as a potential conflict of interest," said Merrill Goozner, director of the liberal Center for Science in the Public Interest. "You want a barrier between the regulated and regulators" (Mundy 2005). Gottlieb argued that his experience as an industry analyst was an asset because it "helped me appreciate where regulatory policy can be improved upon to help enable medical innovation and to turn scientific breakthroughs into practical medical solutions that can help patients" (Mundy 2005).

Shortly after his FDA appointment, Gottlieb was diagnosed with Hodgkin lymphoma, a form of cancer, and underwent successful treatment. He left the FDA in 2007 to become a partner in the health care division of New Enterprise Associates, one of the largest venture capital firms in the world. In 2013, Gottlieb was selected to serve as a member of the Federal Health Information Technology Policy Committee in the Department of Health and Human Services. Four years later, President Donald Trump nominated Gottlieb to become commissioner of the FDA.

During Gottlieb's Senate confirmation hearings, supporters claimed that his experiences as a cancer survivor would make him responsive to the needs of patients. Calling him an "excellent choice," Jonathan Wilcox of the advocacy group Patients Rising wrote that "as a physician, scholar, and also a patient, Dr. Gottlieb has the perspective and ideas to bring great, lasting and transformative change. Patients stand to immeasurably benefit from his leadership" (John 2017). Critics once again raised concerns about potential conflicts of interest, noting that Gottlieb "would wield considerable power over companies and investment firms that have paid him millions of dollars over the years" (Thomas 2017). In response to such concerns, Gottlieb agreed to recuse himself for one year from making decisions involving more than 20 companies he had worked with in the past. He also announced plans to resign from positions at the American Enterprise Institute, the New York University School of Medicine, and the Society of Hospital Medicine. The Senate voted 57–42 in favor of confirmation.

Upon assuming the position of FDA commissioner, Gottlieb promised to focus on a list of priorities that included addressing the opioid-addiction epidemic, expediting the approval process for pharmaceutical products, and reducing the cost of prescription drugs. He also announced a goal of lowering the nicotine levels in cigarettes to "non-addictive or minimally addictive levels" (Gormley 2017). "As a physician who cared for hospitalized cancer patients, and as a cancer survivor myself, I saw first-hand the impact of tobacco," Gottlieb explained. "And I know all too well that it's cigarettes that are the primary cause of tobacco-related disease and death. What's now clear is that the FDA is at a unique moment in history, with profound new tools to address this devastating impact" (Fojtik 2017).

Proponents of vaping argued that e-cigarettes offered a safer alternative to cigarettes that could help smokers reduce the harmful health effects of tobacco use. While Gottlieb said he remained open to the possibility of using non-combustible methods of administering nicotine to help people quit smoking, he also expressed concerns about the strong appeal that flavored e-cigarettes seemed to have for children and teenagers. FDA research found rising levels of youth vaping, along with growing concern among parents and teachers. Referring to the increase in youth e-cigarette consumption as an "epidemic," Gottlieb insisted that "this disturbing and accelerating trajectory of use we're seeing in youth, and the resulting path to addiction, must end" (McGinley 2018).

In an effort to curb teen vaping, the FDA issued over 1,000 letters to stores—including national retail chains such as Walmart, Walgreens, and 7-Eleven—warning them of the penalties for selling nicotine products to minors. Gottlieb also met with executives from the top five manufacturers of e-cigarettes, who represented 97 percent of the market, to find ways to reduce the appeal of e-cigarettes for teenagers. "The youth risk is paramount," he declared. "In closing the on-ramp for kids, we're going to have to narrow the off-ramp for adults who want to migrate off combustible tobacco and onto e-cigs" (McGinley 2018). Gottlieb also issued a public statement warning that if e-cigarette manufacturers failed to cooperate with the FDA to "substantially reverse" the upward trend of teenage vaping, he was prepared to temporarily or permanently ban the distribution of flavored tobacco products.

Proponents of vaping disapproved of Gottlieb's efforts to restrict access to e-cigarette products by adults. Yet some tobacco-control advocacy groups—such as the American Heart Association and the Campaign for Tobacco-Free Kids—charged that Gottlieb was moving too slowly to address youth vaping. These groups filed lawsuits against the FDA, claiming that the agency failed to regulate the e-cigarette industry to prevent its products from appealing to kids. "You're going to see us take enforcement actions very soon against some of those products that we think are being inappropriately marketed to kids," Gottlieb responded, "and we'll continue to push on that very hard because no child should be using any tobacco product" (Court 2018).

In March 2019, Gottlieb surprised many observers by announcing his resignation as FDA commissioner. In a statement to FDA employees, he expressed a desire to spend more time with his family. During his tenure, Gottlieb earned a reputation as one of the few members of the Trump administration who pushed for increased federal regulation of industry. People on both sides of the vaping controversy waited anxiously to see whether Gottlieb's successor would continue to advance his policies. "Commissioner Gottlieb has made several bold proposals that, if implemented, have the potential to save more lives from tobacco use than the actions of any previous Administration," said Matthew Myers of the Campaign for Tobacco-Free Kids. "Commissioner Gottlieb's legacy will depend on whether his many proposals are implemented and, in the case of the youth e-cigarette epidemic, strengthened going forward" (Wamsley 2019).

Further Reading

Court, Emma. 2018. "Young People Apparently Don't Realize These Popular 'Crème Brulée' E-Cigarettes Contain Nicotine." *MarketWatch,* April 20, 2018. https://www.marketwatch.com/story/many-young-people-are-missing -something-important-about-popular-e-cigarette-juul-2018-04-18.

Fojtik, Brian. 2017. "Trump's FDA Commissioner Transforms the Government's Policy on E-Cigarettes." *National Review,* August 14, 2017. https://www .nationalreview.com/2017/08/food-drug-administration-commissioner -scott-gottlieb-changes-united-states-tobacco-e-cigarette-policy/.

Gormley, Chuck. 2017. "Gottlieb Sees 'Watershed Opportunity' to Shape Future of FDA's Regulatory Process." Healio, November 16, 2017. https://www .healio.com/hematology-oncology/lymphoma/news/online/%7B6c 15a1c9-3caa-4875-a4d8-93e3fb25faf8%7D/gottlieb-sees-watershed -opportunity-to-shape-future-of-fdas-regulatory-process.

John. 2017. "Why Patients Win with Physician-Scholar-Survivor Scott Gottlieb at FDA." Patients Rising, March 21, 2017. https://patientsrising.org /patients-win-scott-gottlieb-fda/.

McGinley, Laurie. 2018. "FDA Chief Calls Youth E-Cigarettes an 'Epidemic.'" *Washington Post,* September 12, 2018. https://www.washingtonpost.com /national/health-science/fda-chief-calls-youth-use-of-juul-other -e-cigarettes-an-epidemic/2018/09/12/ddaa6612-b5c8-11e8-a7b5 -adaaa5b2a57f_story.html.

Mundy, Alicia. 2005. "Wall Street Biotech Insider Gets No. 2 Job at the FDA." *Seattle Times,* August 24, 2005. http://old.seattletimes.com/html/health careandcosts/2002450292_gottlieb24.html.

Thomas, Katie. 2017. "FDA Nominee, Paid Millions by Industry, Says He'll Recuse Himself if Needed." *New York Times,* March 29, 2017. https:// www.nytimes.com/2017/03/29/health/fda-nominee-scott-gottlieb -recuse-conflicts.html.

Wamsley, Laurel. 2019. "FDA Commissioner Scott Gottlieb Announces He Will Resign." NPR, March 5, 2019. https://www.npr.org/sections/health-shots /2019/03/05/700482545/fda-commissioner-scott-gottlieb -announces-he-will-resign.

David Kessler (1951–)

Former FDA commissioner, author, pediatrician, and professor

David A. Kessler was born on May 13, 1951, in Freeport, Long Island, New York. His father, Irving Kessler, served as president of Kessler Brothers, a jewelry manufacturer. David Kessler attended Amherst College, earning a bachelor's degree in 1973. He went on to receive a doctorate from the Harvard Medical School as well as a law degree from the University of Chicago. Kessler served his medical residency at the Johns Hopkins University Hospital in Baltimore, where he specialized in pediatrics. He later added an advanced professional certificate in management from the New York University Graduate School of Business Administration.

In 1984, Kessler began teaching in the areas of pediatrics, epidemiology, and social medicine at both the Columbia University Law School and the Albert Einstein College of Medicine. He also served as a consultant to federal government agencies and lawmakers on issues relating to public health and consumer safety. He worked with Senator Orrin Hatch (R-UT) to develop regulations for food additives and tobacco products, for instance, and chaired a committee that advised the Secretary of Health and Human Services. In 1990, President George H. W. Bush appointed Kessler as commissioner of the U.S. Food and Drug Administration

(FDA), the federal agency responsible for ensuring the safety of food, dietary supplements, medications, cosmetics, and tobacco products. Kessler was reappointed by President Bill Clinton in 1993 and remained in the position until he resigned in 1997.

During his seven years as commissioner of the FDA, Kessler improved the agency's public image by reducing the amount of time it took to approve or reject new drugs, including medicines used to combat the AIDS virus. He also oversaw the enactment of regulations that required standardized nutritional facts to appear on all processed food labels. Kessler is best known, however, for leading the FDA during the "Tobacco Wars" of the 1990s. During his tenure, FDA investigators discovered that tobacco companies intentionally manipulated the nicotine levels in cigarettes to foster chemical addictions that kept consumers coming back for more. In 1994 testimony before a congressional committee, Kessler noted that two-thirds of cigarette smokers wanted to quit but were unable to do so. Given the harmful effects of smoking, he demanded "fundamental changes in tobacco policy based solely and exclusively on what is good for the public's health without making unnecessary concessions to the tobacco industry" (Rosenbaum 1998).

Kessler faced staunch resistance from the powerful tobacco lobby and its political allies in Congress. He described his battle to gain jurisdiction over the tobacco industry as the greatest challenge of his time with the FDA. "I underestimated the power of the industry," he acknowledged. "They have their tentacles in government, in media, and the scientific and medical communities" ("David Kessler's Battle" 2002). Kessler's work contributed to the Master Settlement Agreement between the tobacco industry and the attorneys general from 46 states, which required the leading cigarette manufacturers to pay $206 billion to reimburse smoking-related health care costs and to support programs aimed at preventing young people from smoking. The tobacco companies agreed to stop targeting children with advertisements featuring cartoon characters or celebrities, to discontinue outdoor advertising, and to restrict advertisements in magazines often read by children and teenagers. The arrangement also prohibited class-action lawsuits against cigarette companies and limited the companies' liability for punitive and compensatory damages.

In 2000, after Kessler had resigned from the agency, the U.S. Supreme Court denied the FDA's bid to establish regulatory authority over tobacco in *Brown and Williamson v. FDA*. "They just didn't see the fact that nicotine is a drug," Kessler stated. "One of the Supreme Court justices said nicotine is no different from a horror movie. And I'm sitting there—What? Nicotine is a powerful addictive drug, and the justice said, 'Well, you know, horror movies get your adrenaline pumping'" ("David Kessler's Battle" 2002). In 2001, Kessler published a book about his experiences at the FDA, *A Question of Intent: A Great American Battle with a Deadly Industry*. Congress finally gave the FDA power to regulate tobacco in 2009. By this time, though, Kessler had come to believe that the industry should be dismantled.

After resigning from the FDA in 1997, Kessler served as dean of the Yale University School of Medicine. In 2003, he left to become dean of the medical school at the University of California, San Francisco. In this position, he uncovered evidence of financial irregularities from the year before he arrived and brought it to public attention. The chancellor of the university denied that a problem existed and dismissed Kessler in 2007. When the university was forced to release the results of an audit from 2002, however, Kessler was vindicated. After leaving academia, Kessler became a consultant and advisor for private companies in the medical industry, such as Opiant Pharmaceuticals, Keas, and TPG Growth.

Kessler has received numerous honors and awards throughout his career, including the American Cancer Society Medal of Honor and the March of Dimes Franklin Delano Roosevelt Leadership Award. He has written several books about health issues, such as *Capture: Unraveling the Mystery of Mental Suffering* (2016) and *Your Food Is Fooling You: How Your Brain Is Hijacked by Sugar, Fat, and Salt* (2012). Kessler and his wife, Paulette Steinberg Kessler, have two children, Elise and Benjamin.

Further Reading

"David Kessler's Battle against Big Tobacco." 2002. CBS News, January 31, 2002. https://www.cbsnews.com/news/david-kesslers-battle-against-big -tobacco/.

Greenhouse, Linda. 2000. "High Court Holds FDA Can't Impose Rules on Tobacco." *New York Times*, March 22, 2000. https://www.nytimes.com /2000/03/22/us/high-court-holds-fda-can-t-impose-rules-on-tobacco .html.

Kessler, David. 2001. *A Question of Intent: A Great American Battle with a Deadly Industry*. New York: Public Affairs.

Lin, Carol. 2001. "Former FDA Chief David Kessler Discusses Tobacco Battle in Book." CNN, January 17, 2001. http://edition.cnn.com/2001/books/news /01/17/david.kessler/index.html.

Rosenbaum, David. 1998. "Health Experts Oppose Legal Protection for Tobacco Industry." *New York Times*, February 18, 1998. https://www.nytimes .com/1998/02/18/us/health-experts-oppose-legal-protection-for -tobacco-industry.html.

Mike Moore (1952–)

Mississippi attorney general who launched tobacco industry lawsuit

Michael Cameron Moore was born on April 3, 1952, in Pascagoula, Mississippi. As a student at the University of Mississippi, he earned spending money by playing the keyboards in a rock-and-roll band. Motivated by a strong desire to help people, Moore earned a law degree in 1976. "I wanted to be a lawyer because I knew a lawyer was an advocate and somebody who could go into a courtroom and make a difference and fight for people and win," he explained. "That is something that energized me" (PBS 1995).

Moore launched his legal career by serving as an assistant district attorney in Jackson County, Mississippi. After only two years in that position, he was elected district attorney as a Democrat in 1979. Moore immediately made a name for himself by convicting four county supervisors of corruption. After serving two terms in office, he launched a successful campaign for the post of attorney general of Mississippi in 1987. Two years later, however, he lost a special election to fill an empty seat in the U.S. House of Representatives.

Moore served as Mississippi's attorney general for 16 years, from 1988 through 2004. He quickly earned a reputation as a hard-hitting advocate for public health who defended the interests of citizens over the profit motives of large corporations. One of his primary targets was the tobacco industry, which he described as "the most corrupt and evil corporate animal that has ever been created in this country's history. . . . They make a drug, and they sell it knowing that it's addictive. They market it to our children, who they know will become addicts and they know that they will die from causes attributable to tobacco-related disease" (PBS 1995).

Although the harmful health effects of cigarettes became clear by the early 1990s, the wealthy, powerful, and politically connected tobacco companies had won every product-liability lawsuit brought by smokers and their families by asserting that individuals knowingly accepted the risks when they chose to smoke. In his quest to hold the industry accountable for marketing a dangerous product, Moore came up with an innovative legal approach. He got the idea from a colleague who told him about a smoker who developed heart disease and exhausted her life savings to pay her hospital bills. Lacking further financial resources, the woman went on Medicaid, meaning that the state of Mississippi paid her medical expenses. Moore decided to sue the tobacco companies to recover the state's public health costs for treating smoking-related illnesses. Unlike individual smokers, he argued, the state did not willingly accept the health risks associated with tobacco use.

Moore filed a lawsuit against 13 tobacco manufacturers in 1994. Many political leaders in Mississippi criticized Moore's plan to take on the powerful tobacco industry with an untested legal theory. Some state legislators called it a waste of taxpayers' money, while Republican governor Kirk Fordice unsuccessfully tried to block it with a lawsuit claiming that Moore exceeded the scope of his authority. Yet Moore remained determined to proceed. "Nobody had ever beaten the tobacco industry before," he acknowledged. "We felt like we had a chance. We also knew if we won, we might just do more good than any lawyer had ever done in history. Might save more lives than most doctors have ever saved in history" (PBS 1995).

Moore hired a law-school classmate who was in private practice, Richard Scruggs, to help him develop his strategy. When they arrived at their first court hearing, they found themselves facing 68 tobacco industry lawyers. To bolster the strength of Mississippi's position, Moore flew all over the United States and met with fellow attorneys general to convince other states to join the lawsuit. He also received valuable assistance from whistleblowers who provided access to secret documents and research from inside the tobacco industry.

Moore's work eventually convinced the tobacco companies to negotiate a collective settlement with the states. Under the terms of the Tobacco Master Settlement Agreement, announced by a coalition of state attorneys general on June 20, 1997, leading tobacco manufacturers agreed to pay $206 billion to 46 states over 25 years. Mississippi's share amounted to $4.1 billion. The settlement provided funds to reimburse states' tobacco-related health costs and to establish smoking-prevention and -cessation programs. "We wanted this industry to have to change the way they do business—and we have done that," Moore said in announcing the deal (Deprez and Barrett 2017). In 1999, Moore played himself in *The Insider*, a film about tobacco industry whistleblower Jeffrey Wigand and his contributions to the case.

In the years following the tobacco settlement, some antismoking advocates claimed that too many states spent the money on general needs rather than on tobacco-control programs. Other critics pointed out that billions of dollars in settlement funds went to private attorneys and law firms that assisted with the state litigation on a contingency basis. In Mississippi, for instance, an arbitrator awarded 35 percent of the state's recovery—or $1.4 billion—to private attorneys in payment of legal fees (Levy 1999). Although some critics deemed the amount excessive, Moore argued that the results justified the payouts to Scruggs and other private lawyers involved. "Nobody's ever sacrificed the way some of these folks have for a cause that's going to benefit the entire nation," he stated. "I don't think I can say that about every lawyer involved in these cases, but I know I can say it about the ones representing Mississippi" (PBS 1995).

Moore received several prestigious honors in recognition of his leading role in procuring the tobacco settlement. In 1994, for instance, he received the Wyman Award as the nation's most outstanding attorney general, and in 1998, he was honored as Lawyer of the Year by the *National Law Journal* as well as Public Official of the Year by *Governing* magazine. Moore also received the Champion Award from the Campaign for Tobacco-Free Kids in 2003 and the Julius Richmond Award from the Harvard School of Public Health in 2004.

Moore stepped down as attorney general in 2004 and opened a private law practice specializing in resolving disputes between state governments and corporations. One of his high-profile cases involved negotiating a settlement between the BP oil company and individuals and entities harmed by the 2010 *Deepwater Horizon* underwater oil spill in the Gulf of Mexico. In 2017, Moore helped a coalition of state and local governments file a lawsuit against the pharmaceutical industry to recover health care expenditures and criminal justice costs related to the opioid epidemic. Using a similar logic to that applied in the state tobacco litigation, Moore contended that Purdue Pharma—the makers of OxyContin—and other pharmaceutical companies misled public health officials, doctors, and consumers about the risks of addiction and overdose associated with opioid painkillers, thus creating a public health crisis.

Further Reading

Deprez, Esme E., and Paul Barrett. 2017. "The Lawyer Who Beat Big Tobacco Takes on the Opioid Industry." *Bloomberg Businessweek,* October 5, 2017. https://www.bloomberg.com/news/features/2017-10-05/the-lawyer-who-beat-big-tobacco-takes-on-the-opioid-industry.

Levy, Robert A. 1999. "The Great Tobacco Robbery." *Legal Times,* February 1, 1999. https://www.cato.org/publications/commentary/great-tobacco-robbery-lawyers-grab-billions.

Mahtesian, Charles. 1998. "Public Officials of the Year: Mike Moore." *Governing.* http://www.governing.com/poy/Mike-Moore.html.

PBS. 1995. "Inside the Tobacco Deal: Interviews—Mike Moore." *Frontline.* https://www.pbs.org/wgbh/pages/frontline/shows/settlement/interviews/moore.html.

Luther L. Terry (1911–1985)

Surgeon general who released landmark 1964 report on the dangers of smoking

Luther Leonidas Terry was born in Red Level, Alabama, on September 15, 1911. His father, James E. Terry, served as the primary physician for the farming town of Red Level and surrounding environs. As young Luther grew older, he frequently helped out in his father's medical office or chauffeured him around on his house calls.

Luther Terry earned a bachelor of science degree from Birmingham-Southern College before moving on to Tulane University, where he received an MD degree in 1935. After serving several years in internships and residencies at facilities around the country, he became an associate professor of public health and preventive medicine at the University of Texas at Galveston in 1940. That same year he married Beryl Janet Reynolds of Elyria, Ohio, with whom he had three children.

During the 1940s, Terry's career became increasingly intertwined with the U.S. Public Health Service (PHS), the federal agency responsible for overseeing and monitoring public health issues, trends, and threats across the country. In 1943, he began a decade-long stint as chief of the medical service at the Public Health Service Hospital in Baltimore, Maryland. In 1950, he took on a second position as chief of general medicine and experimental therapeutics at the National Heart Institute in Bethesda, Maryland.

In 1953, the Heart Institute's operations (including the therapeutic program led by Terry) were shifted over to a new clinical center within the National Institutes of Health (NIH). Terry was selected to serve as the first chairman of the medical board of the NIH Clinical Center. He held that position from 1953 to 1955, even as he continued teaching at the Johns Hopkins University School of Medicine. During these years, Terry built a reputation as one of the country's most prominent experts on cardiovascular disease. His name also became familiar to members of Congress and other policymakers when he was named assistant director of the National Heart Institute in 1958.

The political connections Terry made during the 1950s have been cited as a clear factor in President John F. Kennedy's decision to appoint him as America's ninth surgeon general in early 1961. Upon taking the reins of the Public Health Service on March 2, Terry proved himself to be an able administrator of the agency. As one scholar wrote, "Terry brought an innate decency and the reassuring bedside manner of the old-time family physician to the task of administering 14 government hospitals and some 200 federal institutes and programs" (Kluger 1997, 243).

Terry played a key role in carrying out Kennedy's promise to investigate the potential health hazards of tobacco use. The tobacco industry, along with politicians from big tobacco-producing states, had always rejected claims that people who smoked cigarettes were more likely to get cancer and suffer from other health problems. But studies conducted by the American Cancer Society, American Heart Association, American Public Health Association, and other organizations pointed to links between smoking and public health problems like lung cancer and heart disease. Terry—himself a smoker for many years—put together a blue-ribbon commission for the express purpose of examining these claims.

The Surgeon General's Committee on Smoking and Health included representatives from public health groups as well as federal agencies like the Federal Trade Commission (FTC) and the Food and Drug Administration (FDA). Notably, the committee even consulted with the Tobacco Institute, the lobbying and public-relations arm of the tobacco industry, in putting together the list of members.

After more than a year spent reviewing more than 7,000 research papers, the committee concluded its work. Terry released the group's findings on January 11, 1964. The explosive report, called *Smoking and Health: Report of the Advisory Committee of the Surgeon General,* declared that cigarette smoking presented such a clear and obvious public health risk that lawmakers had to act. "It hit the country like a bombshell," Terry later recalled. "It was front page news and a lead story on every radio and television station in the United States and many abroad" (National Institutes of Health 2018).

Despite continued resistance from lawmakers hailing from states with tobacco-dependent economies, Congress responded to the report in 1965 by passing legislation requiring health warning labels on all cigarette packaging. Five years later, it banned all cigarette advertising from television and radio. Meanwhile, the heavily publicized report convinced millions of ordinary Americans to take a hard look at cigarettes for the first time. In fact, the report spearheaded by Terry has been widely credited with alerting millions of American smokers to the negative health consequences of smoking.

Terry left his position as surgeon general in 1965, after President Lyndon B. Johnson reportedly expressed a preference for the PHS to be led by an official of his own choosing. Observers described Terry's tenure as surgeon general as a very successful one. Not only did he receive widespread praise for his efforts to alert people to the dangers of cigarettes, he was also applauded for his overall leadership of the agency. In the 1970s, though, investigative journalists discovered that the PHS had been conducting a secret research program since 1932. In the so-called Tuskegee Syphilis Studies, African American men with syphilis were denied antibiotic treatments so that scientists could learn more about the disease. This program, which violated fundamental rules of medical ethics, was ongoing throughout Terry's tenure and ended only after journalists revealed its existence in 1973.

After leaving the PHS, Terry remained a high-profile figure in the battle against "Big Tobacco." From 1967 to 1969, he served as chair of the National Interagency Council on Smoking and Health, a coalition of government agencies and nongovernmental organizations. He also did consulting work for antismoking groups such as the American Cancer Society and companies in the health care industry. Terry also returned to the academic world, receiving appointments as vice president for medical affairs and professor of community medicine at the University of Pennsylvania. In 1981, the university named him an emeritus professor. Terry died of heart failure in Philadelphia, Pennsylvania, on March 29, 1985.

More than a half-century after Terry issued his famous warning about the dangers of cigarette smoking, his contributions to American public health are still remembered. The Luther L. Terry Awards, which recognize outstanding worldwide achievement in the field of tobacco control, are presented triennially by the American Cancer Society in conjunction with the World Conference on Tobacco or Health. Starting in 2018, the awards were presented in three categories: the Young Pioneer Award, the Outstanding Individual Leadership Award, and the Distinguished Career Award.

Further Reading

Finkel, Ed. 2004. "He Helped Clear the Air: Former Surgeon General Luther Terry Helped Lead Crusade against Smoking." *Modern Healthcare* 34 (9): H6, March 1, 2004.

Kluger, Richard. 1997. *Ashes to Ashes: America's Hundred-Year Cigarette War, the Public Health, and the Unabashed Triumph of Philip Morris.* New York: Vintage.

Komaroff, Anthony. 2014. "Surgeon General's 1964 Report: Making Smoking History." Harvard Health Publishing, January 10, 2014. https://www.health.harvard.edu/blog/surgeon-generals-1964-report-making-smoking-history-201401106970.

Markel, Howard. 2018. "This Surgeon General's Famous Report Alerted Americans to the Deadly Dangers of Cigarettes." PBS NewsHour, January 11, 2018. https://www.pbs.org/newshour/health/this-surgeon-generals-famous-report-alerted-americans-to-the-deadly-dangers-of-cigarettes.

National Institutes of Health. 2018. "The Reports of the Surgeon General: The 1964 Report on Smoking and Health." U.S. National Library of Medicine. https://profiles.nlm.nih.gov/ps/retrieve/Narrative/NN/p-nid/60.

Henry Waxman (1939–)

U.S. representative who led tobacco industry hearings

Henry Arnold Waxman was born on September 12, 1939, in Los Angeles, California. Both of his parents, Ralph Louis Waxman and Esther Silverman Waxman, were the children of Jewish immigrants from Russia. Waxman attended the University of California, Los Angeles (UCLA), earning a bachelor's degree in 1961 and a law degree in 1964. After practicing law for a few years, Waxman launched his political career by winning election to the California Assembly as a Democrat in 1969.

Following three terms in the state assembly, in 1974 Waxman sought his party's nomination to succeed retiring 16-term congressman Chet Holifield in the U.S. House of Representatives. After winning the primary, he coasted to a general-election victory in California's heavily Democratic 24th congressional district. Waxman held the seat for the next 40 years, from 1975 through 2015, even as redistricting changed the number of his district three times—to the 29th in 1993, to the 30th in 2003, and to the 33rd in 2013.

Over the course of his 20 terms in office, Waxman earned a reputation as a government watchdog and a liberal crusader on issues relating to public health and environmental protection. He accumulated a long list of legislative achievements during his career. In the area of environmental regulation, he helped pass the Clean Air Act Amendments, the Safe Drinking Water Act Amendments, and laws limiting greenhouse gas emissions that contribute to global climate change. In the area of health care, he helped pass the Patient Protection and Affordable Care Act, the Ryan White Comprehensive AIDS Resources Emergency (CARE) Act, the Waxman-Hatch Generic Drug Act, and laws to improve the quality of nursing homes, require nutrition labeling on food products, and expand health insurance coverage under the federal Medicaid program. "For the most part, those laws have been very important and successful and are now taken for granted," Waxman said of his accomplishments (Tumulty 2014).

During periods of Democratic control of Congress, Waxman served as chairman of the House Committee on Oversight and Government Reform, as well as chairman of the House Committee on Energy and Commerce and its Subcommittee on Health and the Environment. In these roles, he conducted investigations into wide-ranging matters of public policy, ranging from the use of performance-enhancing drugs in professional sports to the faulty intelligence used to justify the 2003 invasion of Iraq. During congressional hearings, Waxman became known for his meticulous preparation along with his aggressive questioning of the witnesses called to testify before his committees.

Throughout his political career, Waxman demonstrated a keen interest in the health impacts of tobacco use. He used his position to investigate the business practices of the tobacco industry, educate the public about the harmful effects of smoking, and regulate the marketing and sale of cigarettes. "Today, we take it for granted that most Americans understand the truth about the dangers of tobacco use and the deception of the industry. The sea change on smoking in our country wouldn't have happened without the courage and tenacity of Henry Waxman," wrote Matthew L. Myers, president of the Campaign for Tobacco-Free Kids. "No member of Congress has done more than Henry Waxman to focus public attention on the dangers of tobacco use, to expose the deception of the tobacco industry, and to enact laws that reduce tobacco use and save lives" (Myers 2014).

Waxman's tobacco-control efforts began shortly after he took office, when he sponsored legislation that strengthened health warning labels on cigarette packaging and extended the broadcast advertising ban to include smokeless tobacco products. In 1986, he organized congressional hearings on the health risks associated with secondhand smoke and proposed a bill to create smoke-free workspaces. One of the biggest moments in Waxman's antismoking campaign came in 1994, when he invited the heads of the seven largest U.S. tobacco companies to appear in nationally televised hearings before his Subcommittee on Health and Environment. Rather than issuing subpoenas, Waxman merely invited the executives to testify. "If they chose not to avail themselves of the opportunity, the television cameras would capture seven empty chairs," he recalled, "leaving the public to draw its own conclusions about whether the tobacco industry had something to hide" (Waxman and Green 2009, 184).

Under intensive questioning by Waxman and other subcommittee members, all seven tobacco executives testified under oath that nicotine was not addictive. Waxman's investigation uncovered secret, internal tobacco industry documents proving these statements to be false. He found that the tobacco companies not only knew about the addictive capacity of nicotine but intentionally manipulated nicotine levels in cigarettes to foster addiction. In addition, he learned that the tobacco industry worked to conceal or create confusion about the harmful health effects of smoking. Waxman's investigation provided key information that led to

1998 agreements in which the tobacco companies agreed to pay the states $246 billion to settle civil litigation regarding the health costs associated with treating smoking-related illnesses.

Waxman capped decades of antismoking advocacy by authoring the Family Smoking Prevention and Tobacco Control Act of 2009, which granted the U.S. Food and Drug Administration (FDA) regulatory power over the content, marketing, and distribution of tobacco products. In 2011, he called upon Major League Baseball to prohibit the use of smokeless tobacco on the field or in the dugout, pointing out that the league had banned cigarette smoking by players in 1993. "These issues affect the integrity of the game, the health of your players, and most important, the health of teenagers who aspire to be like pro players," he stated (Associated Press 2011).

In 2014, Waxman announced that he would retire from Congress at the end of his term. "Forty years have gone by very quickly," he said. "This is a good time to move on and have another chapter" (Tumulty 2014). President Barack Obama praised his fellow Democrat as "one of the most accomplished legislators of his or any era" (Tumulty 2014). After leaving office, Waxman founded a consulting firm, Waxman Strategies, focusing on public affairs and strategic communications in the areas of health care, environment, energy, and technology. He also served as a lecturer at UCLA and at the Bloomberg School of Public Health at Johns Hopkins University.

Further Reading

Associated Press. 2011. "Lawmakers Want HGH Testing in MLB." ESPN, November 11, 2011. http://www.espn.com/mlb/story/_/id/25885766/ranking -worst-current-contracts-all-30-teams.

Cohn, Jonathan. 2014. "Farewell to Henry Waxman, a Liberal Hero." *New Republic,* January 31, 2014. https://newrepublic.com/article/116418/henry -waxman-retiring-heres-why-well-miss-him.

Myers, Matthew L. 2014. "Henry Waxman Showed America the True Face of the Tobacco Industry." Campaign for Tobacco-Free Kids, January 30, 2014. https://www.tobaccofreekids.org/press-releases/henry_waxman_showed _america_the_true_face_of_the_tobacco_industry.

Stern, Michael L. 2017. "Henry Waxman and the Tobacco Industry: A Case Study in Congressional Oversight." Constitution Project, May 2017. https://con stitutionproject.org/wp-content/uploads/2017/05/Waxman.pdf.

Tumulty, Karen. 2014. "Rep. Henry Waxman (D-Calif.) to Retire at End of Legislative Session." *Washington Post,* January 30, 2014. https://www.washing tonpost.com/politics/henry-waxman-to-retire/2014/01/30/c06485fa -892d-11e3-833c-33098f9e5267_story.html.

Waxman, Henry A., with Joshua Green. 2009. *The Waxman Report: How Congress Really Works.* New York: Twelve.

Jeffrey Wigand (1942–)

Tobacco industry whistleblower

Jeffrey S. Wigand was born on December 17, 1942, in the Bronx borough of New York City. He was the oldest of five children raised in a strict Catholic family that emphasized hard work and self-reliance. "My parents believed that children were more to be tolerated," his brother James recalled of their youth. "I always had the feeling how much was being done for us, how much we owed for this opportunity" (Brenner 1996). During Jeffrey's teen years, the family moved to the town of Pleasant Valley in upstate New York. He attended Dutchess Community College in nearby Poughkeepsie, where he ran cross-country and studied biology and chemistry.

In 1961, Wigand dropped out of school and joined the U.S. Air Force. He was stationed in Japan, where he worked at an American military hospital, taught English at a Catholic orphanage, and studied martial arts and Zen Buddhism. After completing his service and returning to the United States, Wigand earned a doctorate in biochemistry from the State University of New York at Buffalo. Over the next couple of decades, he worked at several large firms in the health care, biotechnology, and medical equipment industries, including Boehringer Mannheim, Johnson and Johnson, Pfizer, Technicon Instruments, and Union Carbide. He also married his first wife, Linda, in 1970 and his second wife, Lucretia, in 1986.

In 1989, Wigand accepted a lucrative position as vice president of research and development at Brown and Williamson (B&W), the third-largest tobacco company in the United States. Although mounting evidence of the negative health effects of smoking had placed cigarette manufacturers under government scrutiny, Wigand was excited about the possibility of developing less harmful tobacco products. "People will continue to smoke no matter what, no matter what kind of regulations," he explained. "If you can provide for those who are smoking, who need to smoke, something that produces less risk for them, I thought I was going to be making a difference" (CBS News 1996). Wigand also viewed it as a valuable career move to oversee a department with 240 employees and a $30 million annual budget. He moved his family to Louisville, Kentucky, and even began smoking cigarettes. "I was buying the routine," he recalled.

"I wanted to understand the science of how it made you feel" (Brenner 1996).

Before long, Wigand began to grow concerned about some of the business practices he witnessed at Brown and Williamson. In one instance, he claimed that a corporate attorney rewrote the minutes of a scientific research meeting about reduced-harm cigarettes, trimming the content from 18 pages to 3 pages and eliminating all references to the disease risk associated with tobacco products. "When you say you're going to have a safer cigarette, that now takes everything else that you have available and says it is unsafe," Wigand noted. "And that, from a product liability point of view, gave the lawyers great concern. . . . Any evidence, any documents that show any B&W tobacco products like Kools or Viceroys might be unsafe, those documents would have to be produced in court as part of any lawsuit filed by a smoker or his surviving family" (CBS News 1996).

Wigand also claimed that the company covered up evidence showing that certain chemical additives in tobacco products were unsafe. He noted that glycerol, a common food additive that B&W used in cigarettes to keep the tobacco moist, changed chemical composition when burned to form acrolein, a lung irritant that acted like a carcinogen. Wigand also learned that coumarin, a sweet flavoring B&W added to aromatic pipe tobacco, caused cancerous liver tumors in laboratory mice. After independent researchers linked coumarin to human cancers, Wigand contacted his boss, Thomas Sandefur, and demanded that B&W remove the toxic substance from its products. "I constructed a memo to Mr. Sandefur indicating that I could not in conscience continue with coumarin in a product that we now know . . . is a lung-specific carcinogen," he stated. "I was told that we would continue working on a substitute and we weren't going to remove it because it would impact sales and that was his decision" (CBS News 1996).

In 1993, shortly after Sandefur became chief executive officer of B&W, Wigand was fired from his job. Under the terms of his contract, Wigand received severance pay and health insurance benefits in exchange for maintaining confidentiality about B&W operations and his employment there. In April 1994, U.S. Representative Henry Waxman (D-CA) invited Sandefur and other tobacco industry executives to testify before Congress about the health risks of smoking. Watching the proceedings on television, Wigand was outraged to hear the men assert under oath that nicotine was not addictive. "I realized they were all liars. They lied with a straight face," Wigand recalled. "That really irked me" (Brenner 1996).

The following month, Mississippi attorney general Mike Moore filed the first in a series of state lawsuits against the tobacco companies, seeking reimbursement for the public health costs of treating smoking-related diseases. Despite the threat of legal action by his former employer, Wigand secretly cooperated with Waxman, Moore, and U.S. Food and Drug Administration commissioner David Kessler in their investigations of the tobacco industry. He provided high-level, expert information showing that the tobacco companies not only knew about the addictive capacity of nicotine but intentionally used chemical additives to increase its addictive effects. "I wanted to get the truth out," Wigand recalled. "I felt that the industry as a whole had defrauded the American public. And there were things that I felt needed to be said" (PBS 1998).

To protect its interests, Brown and Williamson sued Wigand for violating his confidentiality agreement and launched a public-relations campaign aimed at discrediting him. The tobacco giant hired a private-investigation firm to dig through his background and personal life and plant negative stories about him in newspapers. "They've been going around to my family, my friends," Wigand acknowledged, "digging here and digging there" (CBS News 1996). This campaign produced a 500-page dossier that accused Wigand of shoplifting, abusing his wife, lying on his resume, plagiarizing scientific papers, and cheating on his company expense reports. After receiving the report from B&W, the *Wall Street Journal* conducted an independent investigation that concluded "many of the serious allegations against Dr. Wigand are backed by scanty or contradictory evidence" while others "are demonstrably untrue" (Hwang and Geyelin 1996).

Throughout his battle with B&W, Wigand received anonymous death threats targeting both him and his family, and the tension led to the dissolution of his marriage. Yet he remained determined to go public with damaging insider information about the tobacco industry. "My reputation and character have been attacked systematically in an organized smear campaign," he stated. But "if they are successful in ruining my credibility, no other whistleblower will ever come out of tobacco and do what I have done" (Brenner 1996). On February 4, 1996, Wigand appeared on the television news program *60 Minutes* to tell a national audience about his experiences at B&W. The story of his decision to come forward as a tobacco industry whistleblower became the basis of a 1999 Hollywood film, *The Insider*, starring Russell Crowe as Wigand.

After earning a master's degree in secondary education from the University of Louisville, Wigand became a teacher. He taught chemistry and Japanese at duPont Manual Magnet High School in Louisville, and he was named Sallie Mae Teacher of the Year for the state of Kentucky in 1996. The following year, the tobacco industry agreed to pay $246 billion over

25 years to settle the civil litigation brought by state attorneys general. As part of the settlement agreement, Wigand was released from lawsuits stemming from his B&W contract. He eventually launched a nonprofit organization, Smoke-Free Kids Inc., dedicated to preventing young people from using tobacco. He also traveled the world as a consultant, lecturer, and expert witness on tobacco-control issues and policies. In 2008, Wigand married Hope May, a professor of ethics at Central Michigan University.

Further Reading

Brenner, Marie. 1996. "The Man Who Knew Too Much." *Vanity Fair,* May 1996. http://www.jeffreywigand.com/vanityfair.php.

CBS News. 1996. "Jeffrey Wigand: The Big Tobacco Whistleblower." *60 Minutes,* February 4, 1996. https://www.cbsnews.com/video/jeffrey-wigand-the -big-tobacco-whistleblower/.

Hwang, Suein L., and Milo Geyelin. 1996. "Getting Personal: Brown & Williamson Has 500-Page Dossier Attacking Chief Critic." *Wall Street Journal,* January 26, 1996. http://www.jeffreywigand.com/wallstreetjournal.php.

PBS. 1998. "Inside the Tobacco Deal: Jeffrey Wigand, Former Vice President, Brown and Williamson Tobacco." *Frontline,* May 1998. https://www.pbs .org/wgbh/pages/frontline/shows/settlement/deal/people/wigand.html.

Jonathan Winickoff (1970?–)

Pediatric tobacco control researcher and opponent of youth vaping

Jonathan Philip Winickoff was born around 1970 in Washington, D.C. After earning a bachelor's degree in biopsychology from Yale University in 1992, he went on to pursue graduate work at Harvard University, earning a medical degree in 1997 and a master's degree in public health in 2001. Winickoff served his medical internship and residency at Boston Children's Hospital and Boston Medical Center, followed by a fellowship in health services research at Massachusetts General Hospital and Harvard Medical School. He then launched a career as a practicing pediatrician, a professor of pediatrics at Harvard Medical School and Massachusetts General Hospital for Children, and a public health researcher with over 100 articles published in peer-reviewed journals. Winickoff also took on a leadership role within the American Academy of Pediatrics (AAP), serving as chair of the Julius Richmond Center of Excellence Tobacco Consortium, which focuses on research, policy development, and advocacy to prevent youth tobacco use and exposure.

In his pediatric practice, Winickoff works with families to develop tobacco control and treatment strategies. He conducted pioneering research into the benefits of offering smoking-cessation programs and nicotine-replacement therapies to parents through their children's pediatric visits. Winickoff also developed CEASE (Clinical and Community Effort Against Secondhand Smoke Exposure), a tobacco education program that is offered nationwide. His research also raised awareness of the dangers of thirdhand smoke, or toxic particulate matter from tobacco combustion that lingers on smokers' hair and clothing and contaminates household upholstery and carpeting. In 2009, the *New York Times* recognized thirdhand smoke as one of its Health Ideas of the Year. Winickoff later extended the concept of thirdhand smoke to push for stricter smoking regulations in multiunit housing developments.

As a tobacco-control expert who has drafted policy for the AAP and other medical organizations, Winickoff felt gratified by the steady decrease in cigarette smoking rates among American youth. Following the introduction of electronic cigarettes to the United States in 2007, however, he grew alarmed by the sudden popularity of teen vaping, which he viewed as threatening decades of successful antismoking efforts. "These products are really creating a resurgence," Winickoff stated. "All the work that happened, all the public health campaigns, the billions of dollars spent to try to eliminate tobacco use for kids has been undone. Now we have millions of adolescents currently addicted to nicotine" (Campbell 2018).

Winickoff attributes the surge in youth vaping to the introduction of the Juul e-cigarette in 2015. With its compact size, sleek design, appealing flavors, high nicotine content, and colorful social-media presence, Juul quickly captured three-quarters of the U.S. e-cigarette market while drawing a significant proportion of its sales from teenagers. "Juul is already a massive public-health disaster—and without dramatic action it's going to get much, much, much worse," Winickoff declared (Tolentino 2018). He accused Juul of intentionally targeting young people in order to create a new generation of tobacco users and ensure a lasting market for its products—just as cigarette manufacturers had done in the past. "It's Big Tobacco's dream scenario," Winickoff said (O'Donnell 2018). He urged state and federal authorities to pursue legal action against the company "for willfully designing and pushing a product that will cause harm to the children of the United States" (Tolentino 2018).

Juul's founders insisted that they designed their e-cigarette as a reduced-harm alternative for adult smokers and never intended for it to attract underage users. Pro-vaping advocates argued that e-cigarettes saved lives by helping people quit smoking combustible cigarettes. But Winickoff rejected vaping enthusiasts' characterization of the product as "safe." "If you compare the Juul to a thing that kills one out of every two users, of course it's safer," he said (Tolentino 2018). Winickoff asserted that vaping exposed e-cigarette users to toxic chemicals. "We know based on Juul's own published testing that these products contain carcinogens," he said. "Group 1 carcinogens—the most potent carcinogens known," including N-Nitrosonornicotine and Acrylonitrile (Campbell 2018). "It's not just harmless water vapor and flavor," he added (Mateo 2019).

Winickoff argued that "Juuling" carries a serious risk of dependency or addiction due to the high nicotine content in each Juul pod, which is equivalent to a pack of cigarettes and more than double that of most other e-liquid brands. He claimed that the developing brains of young people were more vulnerable to nicotine addiction than those of adults. "The most susceptible youth will lose autonomy over tobacco use after just a few times," he explained. "So before they even know they're addicted, they'll first start wanting, then craving nicotine whenever they go too long between uses" (Pearson 2015). In addition, Winickoff noted that nicotine causes permanent changes to the adolescent brain that increase the risk of drug addiction in the future. "It changes your brain to be nicotine-hungry by upping the regulation of receptors in the reward center of the brain," he stated, "and there's some good evidence that nicotine addiction itself potentiates, or increases, addiction to other substances" (Mateo 2019).

Furthermore, Winickoff noted that the lack of regulatory oversight means that the composition of e-liquids can vary widely. As a result, he warned that young people who vape may be exposed to hazardous chemicals or illegal drugs without realizing it. "There are hundreds of different companies. There's a significant and growing market for bogus, pirated versions of each product," he explained (Tolentino 2018). "With kids trading pods all the time, you don't really know the source of your product. . . . It's almost like you're playing Russian Roulette with your brain" (Mateo 2019).

Since the introduction of Juul, Winickoff has treated a rising number of young patients for nicotine addiction. "It's not easy to get kids to stop. Their body craves it. They need it just to get through the day," he related. "I can tell you from anecdotal experience just from my office, I've had a terrible time getting kids to give up electronic cigarettes. It's that young brain and extra susceptibility. They're locked in" (Campbell 2018). Some of Winickoff's patients experience extreme physical withdrawal symptoms. "They have an inability to concentrate and a pervasive desire to use the substance," he noted. "It overwhelms anything else the adolescent is doing. They become annoyed, anxious, and don't want to do anything but get the nicotine their brain needs" (O'Donnell 2018).

Winickoff encourages parents to educate their children about the health risks associated with e-cigarettes, including nicotine addiction, and to convey consistent opposition to vaping. "What the research says about tobacco use, which we can apply to Juuling and vaping, is that parents expressing how they feel about these products—their strong negative opinions—actually can make a difference," he explained. "Kids may protest, but they do internalize their parents' belief system" (Campbell 2018). For parents who learn that their children have already experimented with Juuling, Winickoff emphasizes the importance of seeking immediate medical treatment for possible nicotine addiction. As far as broader tobacco-control measures, he has expressed support for zero-tolerance policies in schools and legislation raising the legal age for purchasing tobacco products from 18 to 21.

Further Reading

Campbell, Leah. 2018. "Juuling: The Addictive New Vaping Trend Teens Are Hiding." Healthline, August 17, 2018. https://www.healthline.com/health-news/juuling-the-new-vaping-trend-thats-twice-as-addictive-as-cigarettes#1.

Mateo, Ashley. 2019. "What Is Juul and Is It Better for You Than Smoking?" *Shape,* February 20, 2019. https://www.shape.com/lifestyle/mind-and-body/what-is-juul-bad-for-you.

O'Donnell, Jayne. 2018. "Depression, Anxiety, Nicotine Withdrawal: Trying to Quit Vaping 'Was Hell.'" *USA Today,* December 27, 2018. https://www.usatoday.com/story/news/health/2018/12/27/quitting-vaping-e-cigarette-addiction-nicotine-withdrawal-depression-anxiety-headaches/2388272002/.

Pearson, Carol. 2015. "Report: E-Cigarettes Can Cause Permanent Brain Damage for Teens." Voice of America, April 30, 2015. https://www.voanews.com/a/report-e-cigarettes-can-cause-permanent-brain-damage-for-teens/2744206.html.

Tolentino, Jia. 2018. "The Promise of Vaping and the Rise of Juul." *New Yorker,* May 14, 2018. https://www.newyorker.com/magazine/2018/05/14/the-promise-of-vaping-and-the-rise-of-juul.

Further Resources

E-Cigarette Development and Regulation

Abate, Carolyn. 2017. "Tobacco Companies Taking Over the E-Cigarette Industry." Huffington Post, February 27, 2017. https://www.huffingtonpost .com/entry/tobacco-companies-taking-over-the-e-cigarette-industry_us _58b48e02e4b0658fc20f98d0.

Boseley, Sarah. 2015. "Hon Lik Invented the E-Cigarette to Quit Smoking—But Now He's a Dual User." *Guardian,* June 9, 2015. https://www.theguard ian.com/society/2015/jun/09/hon-lik-e-cigarette-inventor-quit-smoking -dual-user.

CASAA. 2017. "Historical Timeline of Electronic Cigarettes." Consumer Advocates for Smoke-Free Alternatives Association, 2017. http://www.casaa .org/historical-timeline-of-electronic-cigarettes/.

Conley, Gregory. 2015. "Big Tobacco's War on Vaping." *National Review,* January 16, 2015. https://www.nationalreview.com/2015/01/big-tobaccos-war -vaping-gregory-conley/.

Edney, Anna, Sophie Alexander, and Olivia Zaleski. 2018. "How Juul's Teen Success Attracted Vaping Regulation." *Bloomberg Businessweek,* November 5, 2018. https://www.bloomberg.com/news/articles/2018-11-05/juul-is-so -hot-it-s-set-the-vaping-debate-on-fire-quicktake.

Fojtik, Brian. 2017. "Trump's FDA Commissioner Transforms the Government's Policy on E-Cigarettes." *National Review,* August 14, 2017. https://www .nationalreview.com/2017/08/food-drug-administration-commissioner -scott-gottlieb-changes-united-states-tobacco-e-cigarette-policy/.

Gross, Liza. 2017. "Smoke Screen: Big Vape Is Copying Big Tobacco's Playbook." The Verge, November 16, 2017. https://www.theverge.com/2017/11/16/16 658358/vape-lobby-vaping-health-risks-nicotine-big-tobacco-marketing.

Grothaus, Michael. 2014. "Trading Addictions: The Inside Story of the E-Cig Modding Scene." Engadget, October 1, 2014. https://www.engadget.com /2014/10/01/inside-story-e-cig-modding-uk/.

Jain, Tanusree. 2018. "Big Tobacco Has Become Big Vape, But It's Up to the Same Old Tricks." *Macleans,* January 30, 2018. https://www.macleans.ca/soci ety/health/big-tobacco-has-become-big-vape-but-its-up-to-the-same -old-tricks/.

Jones, Lora. 2018. "Vaping—The Rise in Five Charts." BBC News, May 31, 2018. https://www.bbc.com/news/business-44295336.

McDonald, Jim. 2019. "The Deeming Rule: A Brief History and Timeline of the FDA's Vaping Regulations." Vaping 360, February 11, 2019. https:// vaping360.com/rules-laws/fda-deeming-regulations-timeline/.

Nelson, Steven. 2014. "E-Cigarette Advocates Relieved but Cautious after FDA Pitches Rules." *U.S. News and World Report,* April 24, 2014. https://www .usnews.com/news/articles/2014/04/24/e-cigarette-advocates-relieved -but-cautious-after-fda-pitches-rules.

Ridley, Matt. 2015. "'Quitting Is Suffering': Hon Lik, Inventor of the E-Cigarette, on Why He Did It." *Spectator,* June 20, 2015. https://www.spectator .co.uk/2015/06/quitting-is-suffering-hon-lik-inventor-of-the-e-cigarette -on-why-he-did-it/.

Schouten, Fredreka, and Jayne O'Donnell. 2017. "E-Cigarette Industry Gains Allies in Regulation Fight." *USA Today,* April 26, 2017. https://www.usa today.com/story/news/politics/2017/04/26/e-cigarette-industry-gains -allies-regulation-fight/100939604/.

Sottile, Leah. 2014. "The Right to Vape." *Atlantic,* October 8, 2014. https://www .theatlantic.com/health/archive/2014/10/the-right-to-vape/381145/.

Truth Initiative. 2018. "E-Cigarettes: Facts, Stats, and Regulations." Truth Initiative, July 19, 2018. https://truthinitiative.org/news/e-cigarettes-facts-stats -and-regulations.

Whelan, Elizabeth. 2009. "FDA Smokescreen on E-Cigarettes." *Washington Times,* August 6, 2009. https://www.washingtontimes.com/news/2009 /aug/06/fda-smoke-screen-on-e-cigarettes/.

White, April. 2018. "Plans for the First E-Cigarette Went Up in Smoke 50 Years Ago." *Smithsonian,* December 2018. https://www.smithsonianmag.com /innovation/plans-for-first-e-cigarette-went-up-in-smoke-50-years-ago -180970730/.

Yakowicz, Will. 2018. "Inside Juul: The Most Promising, and Controversial, Vape Company in America." *Inc.,* September 24, 2018. https://www.inc .com/will-yakowicz/2018-private-titans-juul-labs-vaporizer-nicotine -electronic-cigarettes.html.

Youth Vaping

Barshad, Amos. 2018. "The Juul Is Too Cool." *New York Times,* April 7, 2018. https://www.nytimes.com/2018/04/07/style/the-juul-is-too-cool.html.

Becker, Rachel. 2019. "Teens Who Vape Are More Likely to Smoke Cigarettes Later: A Double-Edged Sword." The Verge, February 1, 2019. https://

www.theverge.com/2019/2/1/18206902/vaping-cigarettes-smoking
-health-teens-students-epidemic-jama.

Belluz, Julia. 2018. "Juul, the Vape Device Teens Are Getting Hooked On,
Explained." Vox, December 20, 2018. https://www.vox.com/science-and
-health/2018/5/1/17286638/juul-vaping-e-cigarette.

Belluz, Julia. 2019. "The Vape Company Juul Said It Doesn't Target Teens. Its
Early Ads Tell a Different Story." Vox, January 25, 2019. https://www.vox
.com/2019/1/25/18194953/vape-juul-e-cigarette-marketing.

Campbell, Leah. 2018. "Juuling: The Addictive New Vaping Trend Teens Are
Hiding." Healthline, August 17, 2018. https://www.healthline.com/health
-news/juuling-the-new-vaping-trend-thats-twice-as-addictive-as
-cigarettes#1.

Chaykowski, Kathleen. 2018. "The Disturbing Focus of Juul's Early Marketing
Campaigns." Forbes, December 18, 2018. https://www.forbes.com/sites
/kathleenchaykowski/2018/11/16/the-disturbing-focus-of-juuls-early
-marketing-campaigns/#4f7cc32414f9.

Gottlieb, Scott. 2017. "Protecting American Families: Comprehensive Approach
to Nicotine and Tobacco." U.S. Food and Drug Administration, July 28,
2017. https://www.fda.gov/NewsEvents/Speeches/ucm569024.htm.

Higgins, Lori. 2018. "Your Kids Think It's Cool to Vape at School. It's a Big Problem." *Detroit Free Press,* September 25, 2018. https://www.freep.com
/story/news/education/2018/09/25/vaping-teens-school/1404821002/.

Hoffman, Jan. 2018. "Addicted to Vaped Nicotine, Teenagers Have No Clear Path
to Quitting." *New York Times,* December 18, 2018. https://www.nytimes
.com/2018/12/18/health/vaping-nicotine-teenagers.html.

Kaplan, Sheila. 2018. "Big Tobacco's Global Reach on Social Media." *New York
Times,* August 24, 2018. https://www.nytimes.com/2018/08/24/health
/tobacco-social-media-smoking.html.

Keller, Kate. 2018. "Ads for E-Cigarettes Today Hearken Back to the Banned
Tricks of Big Tobacco." *Smithsonian,* April 11, 2018. https://www.smithso
nianmag.com/history/electronic-cigarettes-millennial-appeal-ushers
-next-generation-nicotine-addicts-180968747/#37DvuPF0vSVtK3i9.99.

Korbey, Holly. 2018. "Schools Respond to the Rise of Student Vaping." Edutopia,
June 29, 2018. https://www.edutopia.org/article/schools-respond-rise
-student-vaping.

Milov, Sarah. 2018. "Like the Tobacco Industry, E-Cigarette Manufacturers Are
Targeting Children." *Washington Post,* September 23, 2018. https://www
.washingtonpost.com/outlook/2018/09/23/like-tobacco-industry
-e-cigarette-manufacturers-are-targeting-children.

Nedelman, Michael. 2019. "Why Vaping Is So Dangerous for Teens." CNN, January 17, 2019. https://www.cnn.com/2019/01/17/health/vaping-ecigarettes
-kids-teens-brains-fda/index.html.

Nedelman, Michael, Roni Selig, and Arman Azad. 2018. "#JUUL: How Social
Media Hyped Nicotine for a New Generation." CNN, December 19, 2018.

https://www.cnn.com/2018/12/17/health/juul-social-media-influencers/index.html.

O'Donnell, Jayne. 2018. "FDA Declares Youth Vaping an Epidemic, Announces Investigation, New Enforcement." *USA Today,* September 12, 2018. https://www.usatoday.com/story/news/politics/2018/09/12/fda-scott-gottlieb-youth-vaping-e-cigarettes-epidemic-enforcement/1266923002/.

Pitofsky, Marina. 2018. "Millions of Teens Are Vaping Every Day. Here's What They Have to Say about the Growing Trend." *USA Today,* December 20, 2018. https://www.usatoday.com/story/news/2018/12/20/teen-vaping-rise-here-why/2239155002/.

Raven, Kathleen. 2018. "Your Teen Is Underestimating the Health Risks of Vaping." Yale Medicine, December 19, 2018. https://www.yalemedicine.org/stories/teen-vaping/.

Richtel, Matt, and Sheila Kaplan. 2018. "Did Juul Lure Teenagers and Get 'Customers for Life'?" *New York Times,* August 27, 2018. https://www.nytimes.com/2018/08/27/science/juul-vaping-teen-marketing.html.

Rodu, Brad. 2019. "FDA's Vaping 'Epidemic' Doesn't Hold Up to Inspection." *Real Clear Politics,* March 15, 2019. https://www.realclearpolitics.com/articles/2019/03/15/fdas_vaping_epidemic_doesnt_hold_up_to_inspection_139751.html.

Pitofsky, Marina. 2018. "Millions of Teens Are Vaping Every Day. Here's What They Have to Say about the Growing Trend." *USA Today,* December 20, 2018. https://www.usatoday.com/story/news/2018/12/20/teen-vaping-rise-here-why/2239155002/.

Selig, Roni, Maddie Bender, and Davide Cannaviccio. 2018. "Juul and the Vape Debate: Choosing between Smokers and Teens." CNN, August 9, 2018. https://www.cnn.com/2018/08/09/health/juul-teen-vape-debate/index.html.

Shapiro, Nina. 2018. "Electronic Cigarette Sales Soar as a Door Opens for Teen Smokers." *Forbes,* October 26, 2018. https://www.forbes.com/sites/ninashapiro/2018/10/16/electronic-cigarette-sales-soar-as-a-door-opens-for-teen-smokers/#3ff135576b91.

Tobin, Ben. 2018. "FDA Targets E-Cigarettes Like Juul as Teachers Fear 'Epidemic' Use by Students." *USA Today,* August 16, 2018. https://www.usatoday.com/story/money/2018/08/16/juul-labs-back-school-teachers-e-cigarettes/917531002/.

U.S. Surgeon General. 2018. "Surgeon General's Advisory on E-Cigarette Use among Youth." Office of the U.S. Surgeon General. https://e-cigarettes.surgeongeneral.gov/documents/surgeon-generals-advisory-on-e-cigarette-use-among-youth-2018.pdf.

Zernike, Kate. 2018. "'I Can't Stop': Schools Struggle with Vaping Explosion." *New York Times,* April 2, 2018. https://www.nytimes.com/2018/04/02/health/vaping-ecigarettes-addiction-teen.html.

Vaping as Tobacco Harm Reduction

Belluz, Julia. 2019. "Study: Vaping Helps Smokers Quit. Sort of." Vox, January 30, 2019. https://www.vox.com/science-and-health/2019/1/30/18203743 /vape-juul-e-cigarette-study.

Blaha, Michael J. 2019. "Five Truths You Need to Know about Vaping." Johns Hopkins Medicine. https://www.hopkinsmedicine.org/health/healthy _heart/know_your_risks/5-truths-you-need-to-know-about-vaping.

Grier, Jacob. 2019. "We Are Completely Overreacting to Vaping." *Slate,* January 29, 2019. https://slate.com/technology/2019/01/vaping-is-good-anti -smoker-bias.html.

Harris, Richard. 2019. "Study Found Vaping Beat Traditional Smoking-Cessation Options." NPR, January 30, 2019. https://www.npr.org/sections /health-shots/2019/01/30/690066777/study-found-vaping-beat -traditional-smoking-cessation-options.

Mateo, Ashley. 2019. "What Is Juul and Is It Better for You Than Smoking?" *Shape,* February 20, 2019. https://www.shape.com/lifestyle/mind-and -body/what-is-juul-bad-for-you.

May, Ashley. 2018. "Vaping? You Could Be Inhaling Lead and Arsenic, a New Study Says." CNBC, February 23, 2018. https://www.cnbc.com/2018/02 /23/vaping-you-could-be-inhaling-lead-and-arsenic-a-new-study-says .html.

O'Donnell, Jayne. 2018. "Depression, Anxiety, Nicotine Withdrawal: Trying to Quit Vaping 'Was Hell.'" *USA Today,* December 27, 2018. https://www .usatoday.com/story/news/health/2018/12/27/quitting-vaping-e-cigarette -addiction-nicotine-withdrawal-depression-anxiety-headaches /2388272002/.

Riordan, Kevin. 2018. "Meet America's Vaping 'Superhero.' He's from South Jersey." Philly, August 13, 2018. https://www.philly.com/philly/columnists /kevin_riordan/vaping-juul-addiction-smoking-cessation-greg-conley -20180813.html.

Sklaroff, Robert, Bill Godshall, and Stephen F. Gambescia. 2017. "Vaping Isn't Smoking, It's a Disease-Prevention Method." *The Hill,* March 17, 2017. https://thehill.com/blogs/pundits-blog/healthcare/324534-vaping -should-be-recognized-as-a-disease-prevention-public.

Tolentino, Jia. 2018. "The Promise of Vaping and the Rise of Juul." *New Yorker,* May 14, 2018. https://www.newyorker.com/magazine/2018/05/14/the -promise-of-vaping-and-the-rise-of-juul.

"Vaping's Potential to Benefit Public Health Exceeds Its Risks." University of Michigan News, April 12, 2018. https://news.umich.edu/vaping-s -potential-to-benefit-public-health-exceeds-its-risks/.

Venton, Danielle. 2015. "The War over Vaping's Health Risks Is Getting Dirty." *Wired,* April 2, 2015. https://www.wired.com/2015/04/war-vapings-health -risks-getting-dirty/.

The Tobacco Industry and Tobacco-Control Efforts

Brandt, Allan M. 2007. *The Cigarette Century: The Rise, Fall, and Deadly Persistence of the Product That Defined America*. New York: Basic Books.

Brenner, Marie. 1996. "The Man Who Knew Too Much." *Vanity Fair*, May 1996. http://www.jeffreywigand.com/vanityfair.php.

Eschner, Kat. 2017. "People Have Tried to Make U.S. Cigarette Warning Labels More Graphic for Decades." *Smithsonian*, January 11, 2017. https://www.smithsonianmag.com/smart-news/cigarette-warning-labels-more-graphic-180961721/#QeiWGOrC7yfSQLjp.99.

Glass, Andrew. 2018. "Congress Bans Airing Cigarette Ads, April 1, 1970." Politico, April 1, 2018. https://www.politico.com/story/2018/04/01/congress-bans-airing-cigarette-ads-april-1-1970-489882.

"Inside the Tobacco Deal." 1998. PBS Frontline, May 1998. https://www.pbs.org/wgbh/pages/frontline/shows/settlement/.

Kessler, David. 2001. *A Question of Intent: A Great American Battle with a Deadly Industry*. New York: Public Affairs.

Kluger, Richard. 1996. *Ashes to Ashes: America's Hundred-Year Cigarette War, the Public Health, and the Unabashed Triumph of Philip Morris*. New York: Knopf.

Komaroff, Anthony. 2014. "Surgeon General's 1964 Report: Making Smoking History." Harvard Health Publishing, January 10, 2014. https://www.health.harvard.edu/blog/surgeon-generals-1964-report-making-smoking-history-201401106970.

Lawler, David. 2014. "From Marlboro Man to Smoking Ban: A Timeline of Tobacco in America." *Telegraph*, November 14, 2014. https://www.telegraph.co.uk/news/worldnews/northamerica/usa/11230175/From-Marlboro-Man-to-smoking-ban-a-timeline-of-tobacco-in-America.html.

Levy, Robert A. 1999. "The Great Tobacco Robbery." *Legal Times*, February 1, 1999. https://www.cato.org/publications/commentary/great-tobacco-robbery-lawyers-grab-billions.

Mead, Theo. 2019. "How Vaping Is Disrupting the Tobacco Industry." Daily Caller, January 23, 2019. https://dailycaller.com/2019/01/23/how-vaping-is-disrupting-the-tobacco-industry/.

Netburn, Deborah. 2018. "Henry Waxman Explains Why It Took the FDA So Long to Regulate the Nicotine in Cigarettes." *Los Angeles Times*, March 16, 2018. https://www.latimes.com/science/sciencenow/la-sci-sn-fda-cigarettes-henry-waxman-20180315-htmlstory.html.

Oreskes, Naomi, and Erik M. Conway. 2010. *Merchants of Doubt: How a Handful of Scientists Obscured the Truth on Issues from Tobacco Smoke to Global Warming*. New York: Bloomsbury.

Robinson, Mark. 1996. "Tilting at Tobacco." *Stanford Magazine*, November/December 1996. https://stanfordmag.org/contents/tilting-at-tobacco.

U.S. Department of Health and Human Services. 2018. "The Health Consequences of Smoking—50 Years of Progress: A Report of the Surgeon General." SurgeonGeneral.gov. https://www.surgeongeneral.gov/library/reports/50 -years-of-progress/fact-sheet.html.

Wilson, Duff. 2009. "Philip Morris's Support Casts Shadow over a Bill to Limit Tobacco." *New York Times,* March 31, 2009. https://www.nytimes.com /2009/04/01/business/01tobacco.html.

Index